Seeing the An
Powerful Technique:

by Adam Ha..... Banning

*"You can't invest a billion dollars in your
pocket unless you first know it's there.
Recognize your angelic self,
and awaken the giant within."*

Who's staring back at you?

When you look in the mirror, what do you see? Is it your future, your past, a nightmare

you once had, but couldn't shake? Is it the kind of person you always dreamed of being?

If it isn't, then what's keeping you from seeing that person, that Angel in the Mirror?

Over the years we all build up a residue on our mirrors, until the point that we can't

recognize ourselves any more. This book is about that residue and how to clean it away.

Living a life filled with miracles is your birthright, But you can't own it, appreciate it, or

even see it until you see your own angelic reflection in that mirror. The residue comes in

many layers, like coats of paint on the wall of an old apartment. The last coat covers

many colors and much history. This is where we begin. To remove this layer, one must

learn to monitor and positively influence ones state of mind.

Contents

1 Creating, Maintaining and Appreciating a Lighter State of Mind 3

2 Confront and Release Negative Patterns, Unconscious and Conscious Choices.....34

3 Faith, Focus, Perception & Reality 53

4 Biology, Psychology & Spirituality; The Interdependent Triad 73

5 Silencing the Panel of Blind, Negative & Paranoid Idiots in your Head 88

6 Seeing Yourself Through the Eyes of Others to Recognize the Giant Within 95

7 Reactivity and Chronic Adaptation: "Who I'm being" & "The being I am." 105

8 Creative Expression and the Permanent Smile 114

9 Five Years Later 125

10 Ten Weeks Later 127

Forms 128

Chapter One
Creating, Maintaining, &
Appreciating a Lighter
State of Mind.

What single factor has the greatest influence on our opinions, decisions and actions? The answer is our current "State" of mind. As a race, our state of mind is one of the most important factors in our successes and reoccurring failures. Politicians and corporate Executives tremble at the thought of what the latest public opinion (State of Mind) polls have to say about them or their companies. In fact, if Gallop and associates were to announce that voting age Americans thought the most important thing an elected official could do was to read children's books to their kids in front of the press; then college political science courses would make Doctor Seuss required reading, and Mr. Rogers would've had a shot at the White House.

When the public's State of mind is one of apathy or individual isolationism, then government's relationship with the people is like that of the sheepherder to the flock. But, when the spin doctors slip-up or the politicians over estimate the strength of their public image; then the sheep turn into wolves, and the herder gets eaten.

In a world where political image and public state of mind are slightly more important than running an effective government; the president might want to change his "State of the State Address" to "The State of our State Address."

Here's what a segment of it might sound like:

"Ladies and gentlemen....Members of the Press. There is currently a great war raging in the Middle East. Thousands of people are losing their lives every single day as this conflict leaves children orphaned to wander the streets of Beirut. US envoy John Wilson has recently gotten tentative commitments from leaders of both sides to meet and discuss a temporary cease-fire. But, there is one issue that concerns me most,....and that is.....you, the American people. What's going on in those 300 million little heads of yours? We've installed applause meters in various town hall Locations around the country, and we would appreciate if you could clap your hands in response to the following questions."

> *"1) I can assume that you folks think I'm doing a great job as leader of the free world? "*

The crowd applause drives the meter to the 50% point on the highly visible score board. The president attempts to smooth his furrowed brow.

> *"2) You at least don't blame me for starting this conflict?"*

Once again, a score of 50%, and a bead of sweat rolls down

the president's right temple.

"3) Is your current state of mind concerning both

myself & the vice president being adversely affected

by the recent outlandish reports of our using tax

dollars to hire Las Vegas prostitutes and purchase

Cuban cigars for personal use?"

With a roar, the applause makes the meter streak up from

70% to 100%. Then with a final burst of audience

participation, the meter registers 103% and blows a fuse!

Trembling, the presidents poses his last question.

"4) Would it make any difference to you if I told you

that prostitution is not only legal in Nevada, but

an important part of their economy?"

The applause meter was broken, but it didn't matter. The

audience was silent.

Both our collective and individual states of mind effect the world we live in. For this
reason, it is of the utmost importance that we remain conscious of our state of mind
and do anything in our power to effect it positively.

Negative Vs Positive, Who's winning?

On any given day, the average human being will entertain thousands of thoughts. From memories, to anticipations, to thoughts that are born in the moment; our minds are constantly in a whirl of activity. But, do our thoughts serve us or do they hold us back? Do they empower our state and mental clarity, or do they promote limited thinking and Self-destructive decisions?

According to numerous studies, about 80% or more of our daily thoughts are keeping us from recognizing our true value and seeing that "angel in the mirror." On the other hand less than 20% of them are positive and productive thoughts. Imagine if your 80/20 rule were reversed. Remember back to a day in your past when you were happy, energetic, and you could do no wrong. Positive thoughts bred positive actions which in turn bred more positive thoughts. What if you could live this outrageously happy cycle of success? everyday for the rest of you life without anti-depressants or costly counseling?

Turning "What if" into "What is"

About ten years ago I was given the opportunity to create and conduct workshops on the subject of "detoxification" with a medical doctor in New York City. We covered the subject on the three levels of "Mind, Body and Spirit.". During the process of writing the "Mind" segment, I decided to do an internet search on the subjects of "Being Present" and "Living in the Moment". Numerous books and studies were written on the subject, but they all ended with the same basic conclusions. *"Over 80% of our thoughts are of anticipating the future or remembering the past. Thoughts that are born of the past or the future are riddled with landmines of negativity. Thoughts born of the present are for the most part positive and productive. Remain present, and remain happy."*

This all sounded like a philosophy class being taught in a Buddhist Temple, and I had a hard time believing that these approaches could ever yield fruit for the average Westerner. So I decided to put these concepts to the test on myself.

First I had to prove to my left brain that most of the less productive & negative thoughts I have are occurring when I'm thinking about past events or anticipating the future. To do that, I created a form (#101 in back of book) that had 3 columns running vertically down the page. The top of each column was labeled. The first was "Past", second was "Present", and the third on the top right of the page was "Future". For the next three days, every time I had a negative thought I put a hash mark in one of the three columns, depending upon where it came from. After three days, I sat down for 15 minutes to review my observations. Over 91% of 1031 negative thoughts recorded originated from the past or the future. Less than 9% of negative thoughts recorded came from being present.

At this point, all of the numbers started adding up, but I still needed to see if a state of being consistently "present" could be attained and to what degree it would increase my happiness & productivity. I was left with what seemed to be an almost impossible challenge to meet; to remain "present". Living in NYC, having ADD, and being addicted to television was like saying, "three strikes I'm out", but there had to be a way. Then it came to me. What do we lose or reduce by not living in the moment? Our senses! So, the more I concentrate on my senses the more present I would become.

I chose the senses of touch, smell and taste, then began the second half of my experiment on being present. For the next 4 days I would respond to a negative thought in the following way-

1) Breath in through my nose until I smelled something.

2) Concentrate on my taste buds until I tasted something, (even my bad breath from the morning).

3) Touch something that I liked the texture of. It was a small piece if velvet that I carried in my pocket.

4) Ask myself if I still felt unhappy about the negative thought. If "no", then record it. If "yes", record it, then repeat steps 1 - 3, and ask the question again. Record my response.

5) Tally all responses for analysis at the end of the experiment.

The process was challenging for the first day or two, but by the fourth day I had created a nearly automatic response to negative thoughts that stood in my way. Before starting this 4 day leg of the experiment I filled out a "state of mind" questionnaire that allowed me to rate such things as "Abundance", "Security", "Self Love" and "Happiness" on scale from one to ten. Directly after the experiment I filled out a new questionnaire and compared it to the old one. In all categories my numbers rose, many by as much as three fold. After analyzing responses from the experiment, it became quite clear that an effective "State Management" tool had been created in the process. My world became a brighter place, and the Angel I saw in the mirror had wings for flight.

Maintaining it

I felt great for about a week and then I noticed that the littlest things would change my state from happy and proactive to anxious and agitated. These feelings would pop up like landmines and after a couple of days, I found out where they were coming from. I realized that certain stimuli in my environment reminded me of people, places, things, or events from my past. Those memories triggered specific emotions, and my mood would automatically change. More often than not, the mood that I would take on was a negative one.

Suddenly a thought came to me. If I've been <u>unconsciously</u> anchoring negative thoughts and emotions to my memories, then what's to keep me from <u>consciously</u> anchoring positive ones to replace them? The two questions I had to ask myself were, "What areas of my life have I anchored negative thoughts to?" and "How can I replace them with positive thoughts?"

Negative Anchors to Ourselves

The first area that I've anchored negative thoughts and emotions to was myself. There were a number of events in my life which pop up when It comes to this subject, and I wrote each of them down. By doing this I was able to review my actions from a safer and more objective place.

In one situation, I was 12 years old and living in a small town 60 miles north of New York City. It was a warm summer day, and I was hanging out with some new friends. We were all arm-wrestling each other, and the competition was really fierce. I had beaten most everybody there, when I noticed that a pretty young girl in the group began acting very friendly to me. We started talking more and she was a real "touchy feely" type, which I didn't mind at all. I had to cut our conversation short because I needed to find a bathroom. As I left the group, her brother gave me a dirty look, but I didn't take it seriously because he didn't seem like a nice guy in the first place. I walked into the forest, used the outhouse, and started on my way back to the group. Suddenly I was jumped by seven of the guys from the group, and the pretty girl's brother was leading them. He said he didn't want me talking to his sister again, and before I could respond, he punched me in the mouth. I was bleeding and afraid, but I attempted to fight three of them, one at a time. The kids were older and tougher than me, so I got beaten pretty badly. I gave up and ran away. They all called me a chicken, and those words echoed through my head for what seemed an eternity. For nearly 27 years after that event, the thought of getting into most any physical confrontation would paralyze me with fear. This type of reaction doesn't do much for ones self image. It was time for my interpretation of that event to change, so every time I was faced with the trigger of "Confrontation", I would still be able to function.

As a 12 year old I had one interpretation of the event, but how would an adult interpret it? The first question I needed to answer was, "Why did they come after me?" As an insecure adolescent, I would say, "because they thought I was a wimp and it might be fun to kick my butt.. I'm the kind of kid that doesn't quite fit in with the cool crowd. Maybe I just attract violence." When I look at it as an adult with a few successes under my belt, the picture changes a bit.. I was a new kid that was threatening the male hierarchy of the group by beating most of them in arm-wrestling in front of the girls in the group. They didn't think I was a wimp. They were probably thinking I could put up quite a fight because I was strong enough to easily defeat most of them. This was why the pretty girl's brother didn't come after me alone, but instead brought six of his friends to help.

The second question I needed to answer was, "Did running away in this situation make me a coward?" As a 12 year l would say "Yes"; but by that age, most of my hero's resembled Clint Eastwood's "Dirty Harry". As a 42 year old husband, father and homeowner I would refer to the lyrics of an old Kenny Rogers song, "You gotta know when to hold 'em, know when to fold 'em, know when to walk away, and know when to run!" Seven to one odds is a long-shot , and with that in mind my actions now seemed intelligent, not cowardly. These days confrontations don't paralyze me the way they used to. Being an adult has it's privileges. It's good to finally recognize that.

Negativity Anchors to our Environment

The second area that I anchored negative thoughts and triggers to were things in my environment that reminded me of the town in Orange County New York I grew up in. In one way or another we all strive to move away from our hometown. Some people say this "Transition" is just part of growing up. That may be true, but if we're not conscious of the way we interpret our hometown memories, then navigating through the challenges of our current environments may be hindered by childish decision making.

When I was 7 ½ years old, my family moved from our 3 bedroom apartment in New York City to a 125 year old four bedroom house, one block from the high crime district in Newburgh New York. The house had three fireplaces, a huge basement, and a finished attic; but it needed a lot of work. So at $17,500 the price was right, and we moved in. Moving from the big city to a town of less than 50,000 was a big change for me. Things moved at a slower pace , and it seemed like peoples dreams were smaller than those of my neighbors in NYC. Over the course of my 10 years in Newburgh none of my neighbors ever moved away. If life was anything like the movies and TV programs I was watching at the time, then when the parents got better jobs or made more money, their family moved to a bigger house in a nicer neighborhood. This didn't happen on my street. It seemed like all of the families were serving a very long self-imposed prison sentence. After awhile I came to the conclusion that somewhere along the line they gave up on their aspirations, or maybe they just forgot them. The fact that they were all happy and contented just confirmed my belief that they were not only losers, but stupid as well.

From my late teens to my thirties, I carried the belief that anyone who wasn't looking to make more money, get a better job, or a better place to live; was a loser. I believed that settling down meant giving up on your dreams. White picket fences reminded me more of prison bars than proper adornment for a house in the suburbs.

Anything in my environment that even hinted of suburbia was scary to me. I got married at the age of thirty and my wife Robin and I were "Dyed in the Wool" city dwellers. Four years later, we had twins and 18 months after that, one of them was diagnosed with Autism. After about twelve months of researching specialized schools in the Tri-State area, we realized that it would be best for our Autistic son Jeffrey, if we lived in the suburbs of New Jersey where the public schools offered the best programs for his needs. Within two months we found a house in Northern New Jersey, and closed on it in thirty days. For better or for worse, we would be suburbanites.

We moved in early spring, and for about a month we just focused on minor repairs and acclimating ourselves to the neighborhood. After we got the inside of the house in order, it became time to focus my attention on our front lawn. I got a couple of estimates from landscapers that were much more than we had budgeted for the job, so I attended a class at Home Depot on "Installing Sod". By doing the job myself, I was going save over two thousand dollars. So I purchased my supplies and got to work.

I started the project early on a cool Saturday morning. I pulled all of the new tools I purchased out onto the front lawn. I took a deep breath and looked out onto the neighborhood around me. All the memories of my youth came flooding in on me. I was once again surrounded by a community of forgotten dreams. As I lifted the shovel to begin the job, It became strangely heavier. But, I wasn't just the shovel. My whole body felt as if it was being weighed down by my new surroundings. After about an hour, I shook off the feeling and started enjoying the progress I was making. By the end of the day I had cleared away all of the weeds. Only a smooth layer of dark brown top soil remained. The next morning I installed the sod, watered it, then sat down on my front stairs to rest and appreciate the fruits of my labor. As I sat there, six of my neighbors came up to me (one at a time) to congratulate me on a job well done. They each shared stories with me about the successes and failures they've experienced in caring for their homes. All of their stories were different, but they all shared a common message.

"Settling down doesn't mean settling for less. It just means taking the time to care for and enjoy what you've got." That day I came away with a beautiful lawn and an important lesson learned.

Negative Anchors to Friends, Co- workers & Acquaintances

Did you ever meet a person that you instantly sized up as a nuisance, a threat, a "know it all", or what ever? How did you come to that conclusion? What made you so certain in your judgment of their character? Chances are, something about that person triggered a negative memory of someone from your past. The new acquaintance unknowingly inherited a negative anchor from an old acquaintance.

One of my experiences with this kind of negative anchoring happened in the Spring of 2000. I had recently been promoted to district sales manager at the vitamin supplement company I was working for. It was a Sunday, and I was in charge of overseeing a seminar for healthcare practitioners in Boston at a midtown hotel. During that day I would be meeting our new Boston rep for the first time. I had been told by the eastern regional manager that she was a real firecracker with a resume that would make me very happy to have her on the team. The seminar was nearly over by the time she finally graced us with her presence. She was 5'10", with long flowing brown hair, full red lips, attractive eyes, and a body that would make many testosterone driven male sales managers ignore the risk of a sexual harassment lawsuit. There was only one problem. Before she even opened her mouth, I could just tell she was a self centered, materialistic, princess. I had a lot of experience with this type when I worked with actresses from the New York theater district. It would seem that my suspicions were confirmed when the first thing that came from her mouth was a complaint about how hard it was for her to get to the hotel. I decided not to speak with her too much that day, and we set up a time for me to accompany her as she visited clients in her territory.

Two weeks later we were both sitting in her car as she was driving to her first appointment of the day. We didn't converse much, and that was just fine by me. Trying to communicate with a self-centered princess first thing in the morning was more than my travel weary mind could take at the moment. We got to her first appointment and she presented the products with a great deal of confidence and skill. She was a real sales professional, and with a little technical education she would do well. We got outside the clients office and reviewed the good things she did, and the areas that could be improved upon for future presentations. She was open to learning more technical information, but when I recommended some changes in sales technique she acted like a real "know it all" and defended all her actions vigorously.

The rest of the morning went about the same way, and by lunchtime we were both starving. We both ordered grilled chicken sandwiches with French fries on the side and a couple bottles of water. I didn't want to talk about work and I wasn't in the mood for Idle chit chat. About 5 minutes into our meal I noticed something peculiar about the way she was eating her French fries. It reminded me of something from my past. Something really funny from my childhood. I started to giggle uncontrollably. She noticed I was laughing at her, she said "What!", and then started laughing as well. "That's it!" I said. "If you had red hair, and those fries were chocolates, you would look exactly like Lucille

Ball in the famous chocolate production line scene. You know the one I'm talking about?" "Yeah" she said. "I love that one!" All of the sudden, our lines of communication broke open with a flood of laughter and funny imitations of odd clients we met that morning. I found out that she was a big time horror movie fan, and extremely spiritual as well. By the end of the meal I was certain that she was the long lost child of Lucy, and she revealed that I reminded her a lot of the brother she recently lost. We became fast friends.

Since then I've used the lessons of that situation to improve my relationships with others, and significantly increase my circle of friends. The lessons were:

1) NO ONE is exactly like anyone you've met in the past, so don't unconsciously treat them that way until you get to know them.

2) Most of the time, people will act the way you treat them. Treat them like the enemy, and they will be your enemy. Treat them like a friend, and you've got a new friend.

3) If you've unconsciously placed a negative anchor from the past on a person, then you can just as easily make the conscious decision to replace it with a positive anchor from the past. When you do this, you will open the most free interchange of communication to find out who that person truly is.

Negative Anchors to Money

Most of the world has negative anchors attached to money. If they didn't, then everyone would be as wealthy as Donald Trump. Much of the problem stems from such beliefs as:

- "It's better to give than receive."

- "You can't maintain your integrity and make large sums of money at the same time."

- "The only way I could ever become a millionaire

    is by winning the lottery."

When these thoughts are anchored to "monetary gains" and "financial Independence", then finding your way to a higher income bracket will be quite challenging. My own experience with this type of negative anchoring brings me back to the Summer of 1973. I was 13 years old and my father was a real estate salesman working for a pre-developed community in the Pocono Mountains of Pennsylvania. Every Saturday morning at 6am we would drive 2 hours to get there. We'd stay overnight at the local Holiday Inn, and head back home late Sunday evening. While we were there, my dad would show clients the available lots, and make a few sales each weekend. I, on the other hand, would hang out with other salesmen's kids and get into as much trouble as humanly possible. For the first time in my life we had money. Instead of my father wondering if he had enough money to get dinner on the table, we were now eating at fine restaurants a couple times a week. We even took nice vacations. Our family income increased by 6 fold, and it was intoxicating. It seemed like life was a dream until something happened the following December.

It was the last night of Chanukah, and unlike previous years, we had tons of gifts to unwrap. We had so many gifts that my mother and father totally forgot about my favorite part of this special celebration. We didn't tell the story of Chanukah. A wondrous story of hope, faith, and miracles. The true meaning of this joyous holiday was simply overlooked. The menorah was lit, but its candles flickered without meaning. When the flames finally died down, no one noticed except for me as a tear ran down my cheek. I began to notice what the money was doing to our family, and it wasn't pretty.

Unfortunately, our family wasn't alone in this problem. Many of the other salesmen's Family's valued money more than integrity or intelligence. When we socialized with the other families I noticed the parents were feeding their children a steady diet of racism, intolerance of others who didn't have money, and admiration for "Superstar" salespeople who swindled their customers for a sale. Was this what having money was all about? I had no other point of reference on the subject. So, I began to believe that "making good money", and "doing the right thing" were not compatible concepts. I was thoroughly convinced of this one year later when my fathers boss was taken away from his office in handcuffs by FBI Agents. The sales organization that my father worked for turned out to be a front for a notorious crime family in New York City. Since then, my ears perked up every time I heard of a wealthy or famous individual being arrested for doing something illegal.

Up until my 40th birthday I had never figured out why I always chose the path of less financial success. On that day I had a long conversation with a wealthy client of mine. He asked me, "What would be the thing you feared most about being successful?" I thought for a moment, and replied, "Loosing my integrity or my freedom." We stood their in silence as we stared at each other for several moments that felt like hours. I then told him the story of the Pocono's, and he said, "The only way to change a negative belief is by successfully disproving it, and replacing it with a positive one. Read about the life of Cornelius Vanderbilt and then you'll understand what I mean."

In the coming months I went to Newport Rhode Island and got a tour of all the Vanderbilt mansions. Cornelius Vanderbilt's stately residence by the sea was called "The Breakers". As the day long tour went on, I learned more about this man and his hard earned wealth. He came to United States as a young man in the late 1800's with $100 in his pocket, and a belief that anything was possible in America. He bought a broken down old boat and started a ferry service for factory workers in New York City. Soon he built up enough funds to buy other larger boats. He then got involved with railroads and was responsible for what would finally become the New York City subway system. As his wealth grew, his projects became larger and more diversified. Cornelius Vanderbuilt became one of the wealthiest men in America, not due to any special talents; but instead, his positive anchors attached to Money, Opportunity, and Hard Work. A few minutes before leaving Newport, I took a moment to contemplate what I had learned from this experience. I sat in Cornelius Vanderbilt's Gazebo overlooking the crashing waves of the Atlantic, and said to myself, "I can change my beliefs about money and work hard to live my dreams too. Integrity and wealth can not only coexist, but create a magical synergy as well. The proof is all around me. It's time for a change." Within 2 days of that declaration, I began to write this book.

Shrinking the "Anxiety Zone"

The gap between your good intentions and the actions you end up taking can be best described as your "Anxiety Zone". We've all experienced it. Haven't you every over promised and under delivered on a commitment before? This type of behavior not only effects the way others see us, but more importantly, it effects the image we have of ourselves. People with cracks in their self-image find it much harder to maintain a positive mental state. Fortunately, escape from this zone of anxiety and self-deprecation is possible with the proper amounts of conscious commitment and focus.

One proactive way to start shrinking your own Anxiety Zone is by keeping an, "Intention / Action / Outcome Journal" (IAOJ). (Form #102 in the back of the book.) The IAOJ is the ultimate "to do list", because it not only allows you to keep track of your commitments, but also make sure the actions you take yield outcomes that will boost your self image.

Intention

The vertical column on the left of each page is titled, " Intention". This is where you list commitments or promises you make to yourself or others to get things done. The golden rule of this column is, "Say Yes Less." In an attempt to please others or achieve rapid success, we may at times over commit ourselves. When we have too much on our plates, "doing a good job" is often replaced by, "just getting the job done". Saying Yes Less, gives you the needed time to make your actions mirror your intentions.

In this same column, you should also write down when the commitment to yourself or others will be fulfilled. If the commitment was made to others, then it's time of completion should be discussed with them. "Under Promise and Over Deliver" is the guiding rule to remember when creating and agreeing upon a commitment's time of completion. If you know a job will take 2 weeks to do, commit to a month, and deliver in 21 days. By doing this you win in 3 different ways.

1) You look like a hero to the person you made the commitment to.
2) You gave yourself an extra week to do a better job and/or allowed yourself additional time to makeup for unforeseen challenges to it's completion.
3) You fortify your self image by appreciating the part you played in completing the job.

Action

The middle vertical column of each page is entitled, "Action". This is where you record actions taken to fulfill commitments. It's important to point out that this is not a strategic planning tool, so don't fill out this section until after each action has been completed. When taking an action, ask yourself, "If this commitment was made to me by someone else, what actions would they have to take to give me the greatest satisfaction?" You'd be surprised by the effectiveness of you actions when you operate from that point of view.

Outcome

The final column to the right is entitled "outcome". This is not where you rate the success of your actions. Instead, it's how both you and the recipient <u>felt</u> about the outcome. An example would be "ME: I really came through for Janet. I did a great job. I came up with some really creative solutions to the challenges of this task. "JANET: She said I saved the day and she called me a wizard!"

Over the years, I've filled out a number of IAOJs. Each and every one of them has brought me one step closer to seeing my angel in the mirror, and living the life of my dreams. Give this one a try. It can really improve your productivity a perceived level of self worth.

Lighten your Mental Load with a "Media Detox"

Did you ever feel sort of lost without knowing what's going on in the news? Have you ever felt that Sunday morning just wouldn't be the same without at least reading your favorite section of the newspaper? Does the evening news on your favorite television channel leave you saying, "What the heck is the world coming to these days?" Is the constant barrage of commercials and gossip about the hottest celebrities making you feel a little unsettled? Chances are, you would benefit from a "Media Detox".

I first heard of this term while attended a seminar on "Detoxification" being taught by a naturopathic physician from Massachusetts . She was both the happiest <u>and</u> healthiest person I had ever met in my life. So when she introduced the Media Detox as one of the secrets to her success, she had my attention.

From what she was saying, peoples conscious and unconscious minds are like parchments awaiting paint.. The way we paint our parchments effects our views, beliefs, judgements and actions. The problem is, most of us don't understand and respect the "Power of the Paint". If we did, would we choose to suffocate our parchments in the blood red paint of murder, rape, deception and injustice applied in broad brush stokes by the evening news or the morning paper? Could we still justify exposing ourselves to all of this negativity if we truly recognized that "Angry Paint makes Angry People"? I think not. But the only way to get people to change is to show them how good they can feel without their media fix.

The first thing that you need to do is honestly answer "YES" to the following questions:

1) Would you survive for one month if you replaced the network news with educational TV or some good instrumental music?

2) Could you listen to your favorite tapes or CDs during your commute instead of the radio for a period of 30 days?

3) Would you skip reading the paper for 4 Sundays in a row if it helped to create a calmer, happier, and more secure you?

If you've made it past that trial, then you're almost ready to begin your detox. Before entering into this 30 day adventure, you must assess your current level of mental toxicity. You can do this by answering the following questions, each on a scale of one to ten.

Mental Toxicity Questionnaire (MTQ)

1) What is your general level of confidence in being able to

   successfully overcome daily challenges?

   (0 = none, 10 = extremely)

2) How interested are you in expanding your base of friends?

   (0 = not at all, 10 = extremely)

3) How often do you compliment yourself?

   (0 = not at all, 10 = many times a day)

4) How loved do you feel at home?

   (0 = not at all, 10 = extremely)

5) How valued are you at work?

   (0 = not at all, 10 = extremely)

6) How appreciated are you by your friends?
   (0 = not at all, 10 = extremely)

7) How important is the acceptance of your views by friends and

   associates? (0 = extremely important, 10 = not at all)

8) How interested are you in learning new things?

   (0 = not at all, 10 = extremely)

9) How happy, Fulfilling or exhilarating are your dreams?

   (0 = not at all, 10 = extremely)

10) How often do your daily decisions serve your greater good?

   (0 = never, 10 = all of the time)

Then add up the numbers to assess your overall state of mind (the higher the number the better). The MTQ will be repeated on the 30th day of the detox so you may recognize the full extent of your improvement. The next step is preparation. Gather together books, tapes or CDs for your commute and newspaper time. Pull out your local TV guide and plan your evening viewing at least a week in advance. Stay away from programs that offer fiction or documentaries that uncover injustice or cruelty. Choose purely educational programming, preferably on the sciences, art, or music. These subjects tend to have a grounding and calming effect on people. Many people who I've recommended a media detox to have initially commented that they would not be able to properly plan their days without local weather and traffic news, which would make this detox impossible for them to adhere to. If the same is true for you, then here are some ways to overcome those challenges.

1) The majority of American's have cable TV. One of the least used, but most informative stops on the dial is the "Weather Channel". Try it, and you'll notice that they don't feature stories about rape, murder or animal cruelty.

2) Certain cable providers offer Traffic Report channels, but if yours doesn't, tune your radio to the local news channel. Get your traffic info. Then turn off the radio.

Lastly, before you start your detox, it's important to point out that certain people may have more of a problem sticking to this program than others. For some, the thought of being "Out of Touch" with what's going on in the world may be more than they can bear. If you think you're one of these people, creating a "Life Line List" (LLL) before you start, can make the difference between success and failure with the detox. The LLL is a list of friends, associates or family members that consistently make you feel better about yourself after you talk to them. Make sure that no one on this list drains your energy, complains too much, gossips, or makes you feel negative emotions after you talk with them. Many so called, "Best Friends" would not qualify for this list; and it's best to avoid these people as much as possible during your detox.

If during the next 30 days you begin to get that out of touch feeling, contact one of the people on the list. And ask them "what things they are looking forward to" or "what excites them these days". This tends to relieve the symptoms of media withdrawal. With that said, you are ready to start your detox. Be kind to yourself, and when one of your less evolved friends questions your sanity for traveling this path; please keep the following in mind. Thousands of "Media Toxic" individuals have done this before and virtually all of them have emerged happier, calmer, and more focused. Remember, we attract the type of people we present ourselves as. Consider this an opportunity to bring more positive people into your life.

Constant State Enrichment:
(what remains the same will eventually go bad.)

Did you ever go into the waiting room of a dentist's office and read the magazines. If it's your first time going to that office, you can always find something interesting to read because the magazines, books, and literature are new to you. If you come back to that office in six months and the printed materials are still the same, the wait for the doctor always seems a bit longer than the first time. In the same way, a positive state cannot be maintained for longer periods of time by constantly using the same positive stimuli, triggers and anchors. Didn't you ever notice that some of the old things that used to make you happy, don't seem to do the trick anymore?

It's up to us to constantly create new positive experiences built upon the momentum and expectations instilled by the old ones. There are only two ways to create these.

1) Do and experience new things that are not currently part of your daily routine.

2) View and experience your daily routine from a different perspective to recognize the miracles you've missed.

Back in the fall of 2001, I decided to do something different and take a 3 day intensive course on "Developing Psychic Abilities" being taught on Manhattan's upper eastside. In the past I had noticed that I could "read" people, and tell them things about themselves that they had not revealed to me, or anyone else for that matter.

On many occasions, I had also been able to take pain away from people by touching them on different points of the back, neck and head. These mysterious occurrences had begun to happen more frequently as time went on. So instead of dismissing them as just cleverness and some form of hypnotic suggestion, as I often would; I decided to see if there was something more going on here than my current paradigm could explain.

It began on a cool Friday Autumn morning at 9am. The course was being taught at an artist's apartment located at a posh Park Avenue address. As I entered the doorman building it seemed to be an unlikely place for such a class; but this was the address, so I headed up to apartment 3B. I was greeted at the door by the owner of the apartment, a short middle aged woman with a shoulder length brownish red hair and a warm smile. She led me down a long hallway. It's walls were covered with emotionally charged works of abstract art. I could see that the artist was expressing deep feelings of rage, sadness and oppression. The lady stopped for a moment halfway down the hall and asked me, "What do you think of my work?" as she pointed to the paintings that surrounded us like a museum of nightmarish horror movie posters. The word, "Shocking" fell out of my mouth before I was able to restrain myself. "I guess that's one way of putting it" she calmly replied, and then led me into a large room at the end of the hall. She introduced me to the teacher. Her name was Angel. She was a full figured woman of about 60, with striking crystal blue eyes. As I walked closer I noticed she was quite tall as well. Wearing flats, she still stood nearly six foot tall. We shook hands and I sat down in one of the many chairs that were placed in a circle around the center of the room. Soon, all of the chairs were filled with attendees, and the class began.

Angel went over the subject matter that would be taught for the next three days. We would learn how to read Tarot Cards, sharpen our skills as Medical Intuitives, speak to the deceased, and heighten our psychic abilities through a number of guided meditations and breathing exercises. One part of me was waiting for someone to call me Harry Potter and hand me a magic wand; while strangely enough, my sensible side was calmly taking in all of this new information, and looking forward to the adventure that lay ahead.

Over the next three days I learned how to read Tarot, and I was good at it! I practiced Medical Intuition with another member of the group and was correct about <u>everything</u> I told her concerning her health. I was even right about the small round patch of varicose veins that I felt she had on the outside of her right leg. When she lifted her long shirt to reveal it to me, I felt light headed and had to sit down from the shock of it all.

Over the course of these three days I did things that were definitely not part of my normal daily routine. After taking this course, I looked at the world from a totally new perspective. I was successful in creating the fuel that would maintain my positive state for many months to come.

The last step in maintaining a positive state is the process of appreciating the experiences so you are less likely to forget them. Did you ever open up a photo album and start to remember wonderful experiences that you had forgotten. As human beings we tend to remember our most negative experiences that leave us in a state of fear, and forget about the positive ones that would allow us to operate from a place of love and security. This rampant plague of selective amnesia can be overcome by spending the time to appreciate these important positive experiences. By appreciating them we are consciously recognizing their value in our lives. If our minds label these events as "Valuable", we will be more likely to remember them.

Appreciation

If you can't appreciate experiences you don't remember, then you most certainly won't remember experiences that you've overlooked. Even though, "over looking an experience" may seem like a contradiction in terms, it happens everyday of our life's. When we spend most of our lives preoccupied with thoughts about the future, and memories of the past; we don't notice experiences, we merely encounter them. Therefore, "being present" is not only necessary for creating a positive state, but maintaining one as well. Frequent use of the "being present" exercise described on page 4 can really help. Once you've begun to notice more of these positive experiences in your life, you should then focus on developing your ability to appreciate them. Doing this requires a small commitment of time and clarity of intention. Interestingly enough, the actions of "Effective Appreciators" are very similar to those of us who pray and give thanks on a daily basis. The ways they differ are in their content, intention and expectation of outcomes. Most established religions would have you give thanks to their God for everything that happens in your life. In that case, your relationship with the creator would only be that of a recipient.. To be an effective appreciator you must recognize your part in the creation of positive experiences as well.

The best time to show appreciation for a positive experience is right after having it.. If you put off appreciation for a more convenient time, then the magic of your experience can dissipate before you have the opportunity to commit it to memory. Here are some questions you might want to ask yourself directly after having a positive experience:

- How did this experience make me feel?
- What role did I play in allowing it to unfold?
- What special gifts do I possess that allowed me
  Co-Create and/or appreciate this experience?

- What other people, places or things played a role in the creation of this experience?
- What message was God giving me in this experience?

After you ponder these questions for a few moments, make sure to give thanks for the magic you possess, the divine path of humanity, and God's unwavering love. Start the process slowly, and you'll soon realize; the more you notice, the more you'll appreciate, the more you'll remember.

This process of Noticing, Appreciating, and Remembering (NARing) positive experiences seems to be one of the simplest and most effective ways to fuel a maintained state of happiness & confidence.

The Thing About Greatness

In a riveting acceptance speech given by President Nelson Mandela, he stated, "We fear not our weaknesses, but instead, the things that make us great.". The exercises in this chapter can be very helpful in creating and maintaining a positive state, but without the knowledge and acceptance of our greatness, the pinnacles of happiness will forever remain a favorite vacation spot visited infrequently at best. I think it's fitting that I end this chapter with the following two poems. The first one expresses how I used to view the greatness inside me. The second one is how I feel about it these days.

"Help"

Help me!

I'm 150 feet tall, and I'm being held prisoner in a matchbox.

I'm so afraid that someone is going to discover me in here,

and let me out.

It may be sort of tight in here,

but the pain is comforting.

If someone finds out that I'm 150 feet tall,

I might have to face it myself.

"Pain" or "fear",

why can't there be better choices?

"VR Angels"

Many angels are afraid.

They are blinded by what they call "Reality".

They feel as if life is not real.

As if there is something more,

or maybe THEY are more.

A vast hall filled with winged angels.

They are brought in as infants.

The unfortunate ones stay until they are ancient.

All of them are wearing virtual reality visors.

The sights, sounds, smells, tastes and emotions

are all pumped into their minds by the folks

at the "Department of Preordained Reality".

Every once in awhile one of them will remove their visor.

Their eyes widen as if they have discovered the great truth.

Then the fear sets in and the visor goes back on.

The truth becomes a forgotten dream.

Every great once in awhile an angel takes off the visor,

Places it on the floor, and ascends into the light.

Humans are angels with the illusion that they are "Only Human"

Greatness must be embraced, never feared.

Chapter Two
Confront and Release
Negative Patterns,
Unconscious and
Conscious Choices

Philosophers throughout time have always pointed out that human beings are "creatures

of habit", but according to Webster's dictionary, we may also be creatures of insanity.

In one of it's definitions, "Insanity" is described as the process of doing the same thing

over and over again, and expecting a different outcome. Most humans have aspirations of

advancement, growth and evolution; but without interrupting our reoccurring negative

patterns, we'd have to be insane to believe we could make those changes in an efficient

manner.

Creating our programming

Negative patterns create programming which allows you to live your life on automatic.

The deeper into this state you go, the more you thirst for change. Yet, the deeper you go,

the more the programming prevents you from quenching that thirst.

The first step to changing your programming is to create an "Environment of Change".

This is a technique based on two things:

1) Physical changes can effect emotional & mental changes. For example Studies have shown that forcing yourself to smile will increase your body's production of endorphins.

2) All change is cumulative. If you make a lot of changes in your life, then even unrelated changes are easier to make. By doing this you put yourself into "Change Mode".

Switching to Change Mode and creating an Environment of Change can be accomplished by taking the following steps:

A) Notice the way you normally walk (your gate) and change it by increasing or decreasing the length of your stride.

B) If you are used to using one specific hand to do everyday things like, dial a phone, eat your food, or hold the steering wheel of your car, then begin to do it half the time with your other hand.

C) Change around your activity

schedule. For example, If you exercise

at a certain time during the day,

change it to another time.

By making changes in these type of "long standing habits", you are actually sending a message to your brain to go into Change Mode, and your resistance to breaking down old patterns will eventually begin to weaken.

Old Patterns

Before we can confront and resolve old negative patterns, we must locate and identify them. One of the fastest ways to do that is by asking, "What is lacking in my life?" Is it love? Money? Security? Freedom? Happiness? Answer that question and you'll know what part of your life you've been sabotaging with negative patterns. All negative patterns are supported by a set of beliefs around the area of sabotage (ie Love), so the next step is to uncover and analyze them. My area of sabotage was Freedom. When I first got out of college in the early 1980s, I had about 5 different three month relationships with women. Between each of these whirlwind romances there was a period of 4 to 5 months where I was dating no one. From what I've heard, this is be a normal scenario for most men in their twenties, and mine was fraught with a very common obsession. When I was in a relationship, the first month was great, but after that I yearned to be free of the other persons control. When I was not seeing anyone, I hungered for companionship &

romance, instead of experiencing and appreciating my freedom. This negative pattern happened over and over again, until I discovered it, uncovered it, analyzed it, and finally re-patterned it. I began by asking myself which of my beliefs supported this "Sabotage Pattern"? To get that information, I needed the answers to some important questions.

1) What attracted me to those people?

2) What emotional state was I in when I met each women?

3) What was so good about the first month of these relationships?

4) What real difference was there between the first month of the relationship and the months to follow?

5) Why did I feel like I was being controlled when I was in a relationship?

6) What freedoms did I think I would exercise as a "free man" just before I broke up with each of the women?

7) What freedoms did I exercise after I broke up with each of them?

Questions one and two: Recognize that "Like attracts Like". When I met each one of these people, I was in a state of "Need" for companionship. Since I was needy, the people I attracted and was attracted to, were needy as well.

Questions three and four: My idea of a "Good Relationship" lacked an understanding of how they naturally evolve. The excitement and tension of the first month will often be exchanged for an opportunity to be more at ease with each other and share more deeply. My inability to accept this opportunity and appreciate the change may have also been reinforced by my subtle disbelief that anyone would want to trade the excitement in to share more deeply with me. In the end, it's an issue of perceived self worth.

Question five: One can only be controlled if they choose to hand over control. It's a choice I made in these several relationships. I made this choice by always giving and hardly ever receiving, in the hope that this would make me more desirable to the other person. When it came to going out for a movie I would say "What would you like to see?". "The Bridges of Madison County", she would say. "Great….Let's get tickets!", I eagerly replied. Meanwhile, I hated these type of movies. After about a month of bending over backwards to please the other person, the resentment would boil over, and I would say things like, " You know, I really hate movies like that. Why can't we see something that I want to watch?!" When you take an objective look at this situation, I began each relationship trying to be someone who would always please the other person. This turned out to be a fool proof way to end a relationship in resentment & bitter words. If anyone I dated in my twenties is reading this book, I'd like to take this moment to formally apologize for my behavior.

Questions 6 & 7: It's hard to take advantage of your freedom when you're not free of low self esteem. The only way to break the addiction of constantly needing someone else to feel whole is by being able to recognize:

- All relationships are interactions, not completion of the puzzle that is you.
- In the end, you must be your own best company.

As we grow up our parents, teachers, the media, and even elected officials have installed images that reinforce society's two dimensional view of "Relationship". If you're in a relationship for awhile, everyone asks if it's serious, and when's the date .If you're not in a relationship, people think you're a swinger, a slut, mentally unstable, down on your luck, or just lonely. With this type of social pressure to couple, people aren't given enough time to get to know & like themselves. If a person does not have an understanding, acceptance, and love of self; then the "Self" that you portray to others will be false. You will attract the wrong people to have a relationship with, because they were looking for the person you initially presented to them. The "False You".

Many negative "Old Patterns" are reinforced by an immature sense of self, which tends to reduce self esteem. Experiencing the magical depths of your "Self" without judgment can allow you to evolve past this problem. Like many other relationships, the one between you and your true self has an "initial attraction", a "courtship", and finally a "long term commitment".

Initial Attraction

Has someone you've known for years did or said something that suddenly made you think about them in a romantic way. The story of marrying your best friend from college is not an uncommon one. So lets take that idea to the relationship that you could have with your true self. Did you ever surprise yourself at how well you handled a situation? How did you react to that? Did you take a moment to pat yourself on the back and say, "It's good to be me"; or did you take your actions for granted, just relieved to get past the

situation unscathed? When it presents itself, seize the opportunity and recognize the
ultimate life partner that is your true self. It's the healthiest infatuation you'll ever have.

Courtship

At this stage of the game, you'll have to start asking yourself if it's okay for you to be
this "True Self"? Like in any courtship, the major question that always comes up
is, "Does it feel right to bond with this person?" In this case, you're asking yourself if
being inseparably bound to your True Self is something you would like to recognize and
appreciate. To answer this question, you'll need to do some "True Self Profiling".
To do this, you:

1) List your strengths and qualities on the
   left hand side of a piece of paper.

2) Ask a close friend what they think your
   strengths and qualities are, and list
   them on the right hand side of the paper.

3) Go into a state of conscious presence.
   Some people call this "living in the
   now". In this state you can more easily
   recognize and appreciate your True Self.
   One way to enter this state is to be
   conscious of how your body feels. How the
   energy flows through it. Be conscious of
   the feelings, not the thoughts. Focus on

your breath, and "Being" in your body. Do
it with your eyes closed, in a quiet
place, or amongst nature. After about ten
minutes, bring your attention to the
lists of strengths and qualities, and
with as little thought as possible, check
the ones that best resonate with your
souls true nature. Trust your intuition.
It will serve you well.

4) Make a new list, just of the ones you've
checked. Commit it to memory.

5) If you noticed that being in a state of
conscious presence allowed you to think
less, feel more, and just be a happier
person; then read the book, "The Power of
Now", by Eckart Tole. It <u>will</u> take your
life to a whole new level.

Long Term Commitment

At this stage, it's important remain as consciously present as possible. Thinking about the
past or the future too much can only help to reinforce your old "False You" and promote
negativity. If you do feel this happen, take a deep breath and feel your body. This will

take you back into the present and dissolve the pain of negative emotions. In the beginning, you will only be able to remain fully in the "Now" for a few moments at a time. But, with some practice it will become your prevailing state.

While you progress in your ability to remain present, it's important to note that your brain is a machine that believes it still has more right to your identity than your soul does. Until the time that you are able to remain totally present and prove it wrong, you will be effected by it's preprogrammed self image. So start reprogramming it now. To your mind, repeated information becomes more factual with every new repetition. Also, the best times to introduce new information to your mind is when it's first transitioning from sleep to waking and waking to sleep. Take advantage of these two facts and begin to reprogram your mind's self image by verbally repeating your list of Strengths & Qualities once as you wake, and once before bed. State it as, "I am _____." Make a habit of it, and your transition from being semi-present to fully present will become much easier.

A high level of self esteem is your birthright, but consciously recognizing and appreciating it is your choice.

Old Energy

Back in 1996, I had the pleasure of sitting down and conversing with a medical doctor and author in New York City, by the name of Mitchell Gaynor. He had recently written a book by the name of "Healing ESSENCE" in which he described a technique for releasing old negative thoughts from the bodies of his cancer patients. His unique use of visualization was both highly effective and elegant in it's simplicity. But to me, the most fascinating thing that he accomplished was to draw attention to this negative energetic residue that builds up in our souls and cells. For the purpose of this discussion we'll call it "Old Negative Energy".

"Old Negative Energy" and where does it come from?

It all comes back to Norman Cousin's belief that the human body is more than just an elaborate combination of biochemical reactions. We are also defined by our "essence", the energy that truly animates us. Some theologians call it your "soul", others refer to it as your "Life Force"; but regardless of it's label, this energy is an inseparable part of you that can be both positively and negatively effected by the energy of memories and the emotions they invoke.

There are two basic ways that Old Negative Energy gets imbedded in the substance of our bodies.

1) A physical trauma to the body may heal, but the negative emotions like fear, anxiety, or anger that were perceived by you during that moment of trauma may remain as unwanted guests. The pain, and emotions may now be firmly bonded to that area of your body. Re-injure that same area, and you will to some degree experience

the emotions surrounding the original trauma.
You may also experience those same emotions at
sometime in the future, and feel pain in that
area from the original event. Either way you
have subconsciously planting landmines on the
future path of your life experience.

2) The second way is by having either acute or
   chronic exposure to intense emotions. The
   energy of these feelings finds it's way to
   specific parts of the body that resonate with
   those emotions. For example, anger and anxiety
   will often store themselves in one's liver.
   Fear, on the other hand, will find it's way to
   both the lungs and kidneys. Worry can
   accumulate in the intestines. Excessive
   exposure to these negative emotions can reduce
   function in any number of organs. For more
   information on "Emotion / Organ Connections"
   you may want to converse with your local
   Acupuncturist or Chinese Herbalist.

Locate, Identify, Release & Replace

Hunting down these pockets of old negative energy can be a very enlightening experience. This process is best facilitated by someone else, so find yourself a "Energy Detox Buddy" before you start, and plan on taking turns detoxing each other of negative energy.

Location

The first step in this process is to challenge the body with an emotion, and feel what part of your body resonates to it. Have your partner ask you, "If anger were to reside in your body, where would it be?" Think of the emotion. If a part of the body resonates to the emotion and also brings up a memory of an event, then you know you have hit upon a

pocket of old negative energy. If this happens, go to the "Identification" stage. If not, then move to the next emotion. Try this exercise with feelings like jealousy, sadness, anxiety, hopelessness, fear or any other negative emotions you can think of.

Identification

At this point, you'll want to give this energy substance by recognizing it's characteristics. You can do this by having your partner ask you the following questions, (It's best to do this with your eyes closed):

- "Where is the emotion located in your body?"
- "If it were to have a shape, what would it be?"
- "How large is it?"
- "What color is it?"

- "Is it heavy or light?"

- "What surface texture does it have?"

- "If it had a face on it, what emotion would it
    be expressing?"

Then have your partner repeat it's characteristics back to you. For Example, "So the emotion is right about here on you (point to it). It's shaped like a cube with sharp corners. It's about 3 inches wide, bright red, and is as heavy as lead. It's surface is rough like sand paper, and it looks really angry. Is that about right?"

Release and Replace

When you can really see it as an "entity", you'll want to release it and replace it with a more positive energy/emotion/memory. To do this, you'll want to have your partner say the following:

"Now imagine that it's hollow like a balloon. And like a balloon, it also has a
tied off point at the bottom of it that you can attach a string to. I'd like you to
attach a string to it. The string is thin, white and about two feet long. I'd like
you to tie the other end of the string to your pelvic bone. Single knot, double
knot, triple knot. You'll notice that there is slack on the string that hangs down
between your legs. Can you see this? In a couple of moments, I'm going to
count to five. When I reach five, a couple of things are going to start to
happen to the object. With every breath it's going to slowly glow brighter
and brighter as if we're turning up a dimmer switch. With every breath it will

get lighter and begin to rise in your body as if it where being filled with helium. Lastly, it's emotion will become more and more intense during this process. Are you ready for the count? Alright. One, two, three, four, five. Breathe in. With this and every breath to come you'll notice that the notice that the object is getting lighter and starting to rise. Feel it begin to rise. It's getting brighter. Breathe. The emotion is getting more intense. Feel it rising up higher now. Breathe. You can see it glow with your eyes closed as it rises up to your neck and then to the base of your skull. Breathe. It rises up just an inch more then abruptly stops. You notice that the slack on the string has run out, and the object cannot raise any higher without breaking the string that is attached on the other end to your pelvic bone. Breathe. The object pulls heavily on the string and it begins to fray. Now imagine you have a large set of sewing shears in your right hand. Bring the shears up to the string, and on the count of three you will snip the string and the object will shoot out of the top of you head, never to return. Ready? One, Two, Three, SNIP! Feel it shoot out of the top of your head and disintegrate as it hits the air above you. Now immediately focus your thoughts on the area of your body that once held that emotion. Fill that empty area with an emotion and memory that is the antithesis of the ones that you just got rid of. When you can see that memory for at least 5 seconds, you can open your eyes."

When I first heard of this technique, I must admit, I had some doubts. But after using it with hundreds of people over the past three years, my doubts have been pleasantly replaced with a great deal of confidence in this approach. For many, it's proven to be the turning point in their emotional and spiritual evolution.

The Past does not equal the Future.

When I was in my early twenties I handed my resume across a desk to an executive at a company I wanted to work for. She looked at it and told me that I was a "Job Hopper", and that I would probably not amount to anything in life. Mind you, she didn't even speak with me. She Just looked at my resume. I was pretty flustered as I left her office. In retrospect, I should have thanked my lucky stars that I would never work for someone like that. But from that point forward, I learned an important lesson. A Mind that believes, "The past equals the future" cannot conceive the inevitability of change or embrace the hope for a brighter future.

Our culture has constantly created and reinforcing sayings like, "Once a liar, always a liar", "He's got a record a mile long" and "You can't teach an old dog new tricks". The more we use sayings like these, the more we ignore a simple truth. "The past will never equal the future" unless you live life in such an unconscious state as to consistently repeat ALL of your childhood habits and patterns. This may sound like an oxymoron, but "the only universal constant is Change." Recognize this and your future can be filled with hope and opportunity.

Walking the Walk

Did you ever wonder why the employees of a company follow their CEO's directives. Is it because he has the largest executive office on the penthouse floor or the fancy Ivy League school he graduated from. Maybe because the door to their office is made of teakwood and their name and position are hand carved on it's surface, as opposed to the other executives that only have the standard "Self Stick" bronze colored name plates. Is it just because they're afraid of loosing their jobs; or maybe it's something more permanent, more powerful. Something that resides firmly inside the CEO. This very special something that shines forth in every action they take and word they speak. From a major business decision to the way they walk down an office corridor. It's unmistakable. They walk like a CEO.

What do you want to be in life? How do you walk? Do you notice an incongruency? There is no time better than right now to start walking the walk of your dreams. It doesn't require a fancy advanced degree from a big name private school. The highly acclaimed television news correspondent, Peter Jennings, never even went to college. Most people don't even know that, and if they do, it still doesn't matter; because Peter Jennings has the walk.

Get up and take a walk outside. While you're seeing the sites, ask yourself what a leader, philosopher, or general might walk like. Pick the person in you that's dying to get out and let them walk their walk. When I did, this a highly visible teacher and counselor came out. The gate of my walk became more consistent and secure. My posture improved. As I walked further, I noticed that lots of people were looking at me and when our eyes met I was always greeted with a warm smile. It was easy to start talking with people who were previously complete strangers. This experience left me with a couple of undeniable truths.

- People are attracted to you when you walk the walk of your dreams.
- People can sense your frustration and lack of grounding when you don't.
- You can only dream of becoming someone that you already are, but may have not truly expressed yet.

The Fallacy: Only Accomplished experts can teach

Can a mailroom clerk give valid advice on corporate investments to the CEO of his company? Can a divorced man be an expert on how to preserve a happy marriage? Are a Wiseman's words less than credible if they are not accompanied by a post graduate degree in philosophy. Is our need for qualifications from the people we take non-technical advise from based upon our distrust in others, or our distrust in our own god given ability to discern truth from deceptive illusion. Haven't you ever heard an expert on a subject state their views and you felt compelled to disagree with them? Who are you to disagree with the expert! Fear not…there are NO experts on the subjects of truth and wisdom. When you attended college, did you ever see a class called "Truth 101"? Are there advanced degrees on the Subjects of "discernment" and "wisdom?" NO, but there certain people who are really good at it. What's their secret? They believe in their ability to hear truth, and they're not afraid to speak it as well. The time is now to "Listen for Truth", "Tell your Truth", and Teach it as well.

"Accomplishments" or Irrelevant Benchmarks

A man traveled down a road. The sign ahead read "400 miles to Perfection". He smiles and mutters to himself, "Perfection, Yeah, It's gonna be great", his car breaks down in a little one horse town that's barely more than a pit-stop on the road of life. The car is towed to the local garage, and the man went to the diner and slowly worked his way through a steak dinner. He gets the check. Reaches into his back pocket for his wallet, and realizes "It's not there!" All his money! All his credit cards! His Identification! All gone! He tells the man at the diner of his unfortunate situation. At that very moment the cook comes running out of the kitchen, slams his apron down on the table, and yells, "I quit! This place is a dump!" The owner of the diner looks at the wallet-less traveler and says, "Can ya cook?" The traveler puts on the apron. Goes into the kitchen and begins preparing meals. The evening goes on and with every meal he cooks the owner gets another complement on the creations of his new chef. The diner starts drawing customers from as far away as California. The chef becomes a celebrity. In a moment of insecurity the owner offers his new chef a sizable raise to make sure he sticks around for awhile. The man takes off his apron, walks out into the dining area, and stares out the window. It's night-time, and the street light illuminates the sign the new chef first saw when he was traveling through town. "400 miles to perfection". He muttered to himself, "Perfection, yeah, it's gonna be great". He left the diner. Got in his car, and resumed his trek down the road of anticipation. In a few hours he forgot about his culinary successes, and only lived for the moment that he would enter perfection. He's still traveling that road.

Paths are real. Destinations are often little more than an illusion. Putting off life until achievements are attained will always yield a state of unrelenting want. To Measure your life solely by achievements requires you to abandon the miracles of the moment and live life in the past.

How you walk the path is of greater value.

Chapter Three
Faith, Focus, Perception & Reality

P ygmalion was a mythical King of Cyprus who carved an ivory statue of a maiden. He

named it "Galatea" and fell in love with it. He believed with his heart and soul that it was

his perfect woman. For him, this belief became his reality. One of the timeless morals of

this story was:

"Beliefs manifest reality. Positive AND Negative.

Manifestation does not discriminate."

The "Pygmalion Effect"

Charlie Black was a 13 year old boy who had been kicked out of 6 private schools in the

past two years ever since he lost his mother in a fire. He now lives with his dad in a

one bedroom apartment. His last six teachers have labeled him a trouble maker and have

all stated openly that right from the beginning they "just didn't trust him." Every day

after dismissal, Charlie would spend about a half hour talking to his friends in the woods

behind the school. All of the others would smoke pot and cigarettes back there, but

Charlie would always abstain. He may have never smoked or drank, but he was labeled

a "Pothead" by the teachers who would see him heading back into the woods after school

each day.

After about 30 minutes with his friends, Charlie would always say, "Gotta Go..", and he would head out of the woods, through the abandoned junkyard, and down a road toward the less savory part of town. As his friends watched him leave, one of them would always say something like, "Damn...what part of the slums does he live in?"

One chilly afternoon in March, the sound of police sirens broke the misty silence of the forest behind the school. The teachers watched from the classroom windows as four police officers led two dozen or so students out of the forest and towards the school. They were met in front of the school by the Principal, both Assistant Principals, and three guidance counselors. After a moment, the principal shook hands with two of the officers. The police left, and the counselors led the students back to the school.

By the next day, 3 of the students were expelled, 12 suspended, and now it was Charlie's turn to explain himself to Mr. Donald Wurtmore, the Assistant Principal. One of the guidance counselors escorted Charlie to Mr. Wurtmore's office and sat him down in a small wooden chair in front of the assistant principal's large gray metal desk. Mr. Wurtmore came in and instead of sitting down in his big leather chair behind the desk, he pulled out a folding metal chair from behind the door; placed it in front of Charlie and sat down. He leaned forward so his face was no more than a foot away from Charlie's and said, "So what are we going to do with you...Huh?"

Charlie was quiet, but maintained eye contact because he knew this was serious."Some students around here seem to think that drinking beer and smoking pot on school property is the IN thing to do." Wurtmore sternly whispered. "BUT!!! Until I'm notified to the contrary; it is ILLEGAL for a thirteen year old to consume beer, and ANYONE to smoke pot! Do you know how close you were to being in big trouble with the police?! I will not have your issues with substance abuse embarrass and threaten the reputation of this school. Can you give me one good reason why I shouldn't expel you this very second?" In a nervous yet certain tone Charlie replied, "I don't drink beer, and I don't even smoke cigarettes, never mind pot. I was just back there hanging out with my friends, like I do everyday after school."

"Why do I find that extremely hard to believe???? Could it be the six schools you've been thrown out of in the past 2 years? Or maybe the fact that every one of your teachers that I've had the opportunity to talk with in the past day have labeled you as a TROUBLEMAKER and a RAPSHEET just waiting to be written!!!??"

Charlie took a deep breath and replied, "I don't drink. I don't smoke, and I'm not a liar. Mr. Wurtmore....Please...You've got to believe me!"
The assistant principal stared into Charlie's eyes for what seemed an eternity. Wurtmore thought, "Could this kid be telling the truth? He really seems sincere. But what about his history? Was he really that good a lair?" Then Wurtmore replied, "You MAY be looking for school number seven after tomorrow, but until that time, I've got some thinking to do. Now get out of my office and get back to class!"

For the rest of the day the dilemma of "what to do with Charlie Black" was foremost in the thoughts of Assistant Principal Wurtmore. Donald knew he needed some wisdom and insightful advice on this issue, and his old friend Father Garity was the right man for the job. Many years back he would visit him at his church on the other side of town.

"Father Garity always had a special way of looking at things", they would say. "He always saw the miracles that other people missed."

After school Donald went to visit Father Garity at the church. When he walked in the father was speaking with a group of teenage volunteers who were carrying pots and pans to the church's soup kitchen next door. Father Garity looked up and spotted him coming in. "Well…If it isn't Donald Wurtmore, my old friend. Lad.. Where ya bin hidin yer self?" Donald and Father Garity gave each other a stiff embrace and both headed to the parish office in the rear of the church. They sat face to face in the father's office, and Garity asked, "So what brings you to my house of lost angels?"

"I need your advise, Father."

"What's on your mind, Donald?"

"There's this student at the high school that I have to make a decision about."

"A Decision?" replied Father Garity

"Yes….To expel him or not."

"Well…What's he done wrong?"

"Principal James and I have reason to believe that he was one of a group of students that was smoking pot and drinking beer behind the school yesterday."

"Reason to believe?" inquired Father Garity.

"Yes. He's been labeled a troublemaker by the last 6 schools he was kicked out of, and he was seen hanging out behind the school with known marijuana users in the past."

"So if you're so sure he did it , then why are you talking to me about it? I mean I'm glad to see you, but I'm just wondering."

"Well Father….When I confronted the boy about it, he denied it with such great sincerity that I almost wanted to believe him. But he IS a troublemaker. His record clearly

shows that. I just don't know what to think, Father."

"Donald, People often become who you believe they are. Let me tell you about a young

boy who came to our parish about a year ago. He was only 12 at the time, and his father

brought him in on a Sunday for services. Afterwards, his dad introduced him to me and

for some reason, the three of us really hit it off. In retrospect, I guess I saw something

special and genuine in the boy, and he appreciated my recognizing it. The very next week

he showed up as a volunteer to help out at our new soup kitchen. His enthusiasm was

contagious, and after about a month this young lad was running the program with teens

five years his senior gladly taking orders from him. He's also been an invaluable asset in

our fundraising efforts as well. Personally I think he's after my job, and if I didn't love

him so much, I'd probably run him out of town. The point is, when I first met the boy, his

father was concerned that he was heading down the wrong path in life, but instead of me

labeling him as a juvenile delinquent, I took the time to see him for the special person he

was. He became who I really knew he was. Donald, I think it might be good if you met

the boy. How 'bout it?"

"Sure Father, This kid sounds like a breath of fresh air."

Father Garity picks up his phone, dialed the extension for the soup kitchen and said,

"Marion, could tell our little general down there that I'd like him to meet someone in my

office."

A few moments went bye. Then there's a knock at the door and it opens.

"Donald Wurtmore.....I'd like to introduce you to the brains

and heart behind our Soup Kitchen."

There, in the doorway stood Charlie Black.

We all know a Charlie Black, but do we know him or are we "creating" him through our judgments. You take a man. Hand him a rifle, and stick him in the jungle. He becomes a hunter. If you take that same man and stick him in a cage, he becomes the wild animal now hunted by others. Studies have proven the existence of the "Pygmalion Effect". One of the classic pieces of research was conducted in a number of junior high schools around America. Teachers were told that their classes consisted of two groups of students; "advanced super achievers" and "troubled underachievers" who were bused in from another district. This was false information. All the members of each class were hand selected to all have approximately the same IQ, Grade Point Averages, and social temperament. If the Pygmalion Effect was a myth, then all the students would have approximately the same grades at the end of the year. This was not the case in any of the classes studied.

Four main observations were consistently reported during these studies. They were:

1) The children that were labeled "Troubled Underachievers" scored consistently in the lower half of grades in each class.

2) Those who were given the label of "Super Achievers" consistently scored in the upper half of grades in each class.

3) The lions share of disruptive activity in the class was started by the students labels "Troubled Underachievers".

4) The majority of students labeled "Super Achievers" scored

significantly higher grades than ever before.

The student's tests were standardized. The scoring of these tests could not be effected by teacher subjectivity. All questions were "True/False", "Yes/No", or multiple choice. There was no doubt about it . The "Pygmalion Effect" exists. The teachers thought that each of their classes were had good & bad students, and even though this was not the truth, it became so.

We thought the effects of prejudice against blacks, Jews, Muslims, or anyone else simply led to the mistreatment of A group of people. With the verification of the "Pygmalion Effect" we also know that "Mistreatment" created by "Mistruths", can also bring about "Miscreation". If you think & treat someone as if they were lazy, cheap, or a terrorist for long enough, they'll end up proving you right. If you're on the receiving end of those mistruths it can lead to low self esteem, which will negatively influence your actions and decision making. Once again, "Miscreation"; but in this case it's happening to you.

Turning negative expectations into faith in the positive

So, was Pygmalion the devil incarnate? Is there only a dark side to this "effect"? Heavens no! Remember the students who had gotten grades that were much higher than they had ever gotten. Their previously false label of "Super achiever" played an important role in their success. We can bring light to the dark side of Pygmalion by refocusing our beliefs on the positive.

It all starts with thinking of your thoughts or truths as the light shed by either a spotlight, a flashlight, or a lantern. Imagine you've been blindfolded, and brought to a large room in what might be a house, but you're not sure because the blindfold was not removed until you were sat down in a comfortable armchair and the room was pitch dark. A voice comes from the darkness, "Just stay in the chair, and DON'T get up." While you're sitting there, you see the illumination of a spotlight on the wall in front of you. It reveals a circular area only 18 inches wide. Everything around it is still pitch black. The voice from the darkness poses the question, "What type of man lives in this house?" You look at the lit area on the wall and see a section of what seems to be a bookshelf. The books have titles like "The Nazi Movement: Past, Present, & Future", "The Life and Times of Adolph Hitler", and "White Supremacy and the New World Order." You think for a moment, only to hear the voice repeat, "What type of man lives in this house? Tell me now!" You nervously reply, "He seems to have an interest in history, like world war two. He might empathize with Nazi's or White Supremacists. I don't know?!" The light goes out, and another one just like it appears on the wall to your left. Once again, the light fell on another section of bookshelf. These titles read, "A whimper in the darkness; A Journal of Hitler's Experiments on Concentration Camp Children", "The Machiavelli Paradigm", "Principles of Dissection and Embalming". You start thinking, "Who ever lives here is probably not the type of guy that you would trust your wife and kids with" The voice barks out again, "Who is this man? Do you trust him? What are his intentions?" You respond more quickly this time, "If this guys choice of books is any indication of...." The voice abruptly interrupts, "Answer My Questions!!!" You take a quick breath and respond, "He's probably a monster... a butcher waiting to happen!" The voice calmly responds, "WAITING to happen?" This puts a chill down your spine. Are you sitting in the next Jeffrey Daumer's Living room? Are you ever going to make it back in one piece to see your wife and family again? If you do make it out, how could you possibly turn your back on the fact that you know this guys horrifying secret? The light goes out and reappears near the ceiling to the right. Once again, more books. This time your afraid to read the titles, but a nervous sense of morbid curiosity kicks in and you squint to make out three more of them. "Secrets bomb making and demolition of large structures", "A guided tour and schematic of Chicago's Sears Tower", and "Interview with members of the North American Man Boy Love Association." You're an American and a father of two young boys. The fear that you felt two minutes ago has quickly shifted to anger. The voice says, "What are his intentions, and what do YOU intend to do about it?" Without thinking you blurt out, "This bastard's got to be stopped. We've gotta bring this guy down!!" Suddenly, the light disappears and reappears on a coffee table right in front of you. On the table is a revolver, and before you have a moment to think, the voice shouts, "Watch out! He's coming to get you!" In the shadows you see a figure of a man carrying a club and quickly advancing towards you. You pick up the gun, fire it at him, and the man hits the floor. You scramble to find a light switch on the wall. The lights go on. You're in the neighborhood bookstore and a security guard is laying dead at your feet.

When you apply this story to everyday life, the "voice" stands for the influence that the media and other people have in shaping your "Truths" about yourself and others. The spotlight symbolizes myopic and reactive points of view about people or groups of people. The man who was quickly advancing towards you with a club in his hand is the threat you created by believing their was a threat. One of the morals of this story is, "Merely listening to the voice and watching the spotlight will often create mistruths that closely resemble your darkest fears."

Instead, think of the lantern, the flashlight, and the spotlight as tools that are under your control. Find someone you dislike or are afraid of. Identify your "truths" about them. List them. Even write them down. Now think of this information as if it were a spotlight on the wall; only offering limited data about that person. There's more to this person's story. Aren't you curious? Pull out your flashlight and shed a wider beam of light on this individual. This can be achieved by starting a "Focused Conversation" with them. This communication technique has been most frequently used by professional salespeople to access a clients needs, but in this situation you can use it to obtain a better understanding of people.

Think of yourself as a TV interviewer whose job is to reveal the more positive aspects of the person you're interviewing. Keep the conversation focused on questions like:

- "So, what are you doing these days that really excites you?"
- "You look great! What's your secret?" (Don't ask this one unless you believe there's something admirable about their appearance. People can sense insincerity.)
- "So, what do you do for fun on your downtime?"

Remain open to the possibility that you could be pleasantly surprised by their answers. Dale Carnegie once said, "Peoples favorite topic of conversation is usually themselves."

So, let them talk and you keep asking "What" and "How" questions.
Two things to watch out for during this process are:

1) To many questions starting with the word "Why" can easily make your focused conversation feel like an interrogation.

2) The negative things we see in others that bother us the most may be the traits we share with them. Try To be open to this.

During the focused conversation you should also take your body language into account. Studies have shown that mirroring the person's body position and slightly tilt your head to the left while you listen to them talk will put the other person at ease. Do this, and they'll be more likely to reveal themselves to you.

Also, if the person says something of interest like a quote, book title or a piece of useful info; don't be afraid to pull out a pad and take notes. You will not only be able to retain the info, but more importantly, you'll be paying a major compliment to the person. Your note taking has now elevated them to the level of teacher or mentor. When properly used, "note taking" can help to erase any hesitations that the other person may have in communicating with you.

After about 15 minutes into the conversation, you'll notice that your flashlight has turned into a lantern, and you now may be looking at this person in a different and more well informed light. Stay very present with the process, because attaining and maintaining the next step will be essential to your success.

Finally, you'll begin focusing on only the positive aspects of this person. Ask yourself how you might treat a person who's dominant characteristics are the ones you're now focusing on. Attempt to envision them as this person. As you become more successful at this, you'll notice that the way you speak with them will begin to change. You might notice that the conversation has become more interesting. You'll not only pay more attention to the words that are being said to you, but your words and thoughts may be expressed more clearly as well. Compare the way most people converse with a homeless person, to the way they talk to someone of their same or higher social status. You'll see similar changes. So remember, have faith, and focus on the positive.

What do we expect in the course of our existence.

Now lets talk about the expectations we have for ourselves. Take a tally of your dreams, and ask yourself which ones you think are "really" going to come true. The more negative mistruths you have about yourself, the lower your self confidence, the less dreams you believe will come true.

Calculating your "Confidence Quotient" (CQ) can be a very enlightening experience that will provide you with a baseline to measure future growth by. Figuring out your CQ is as simple as:

1) Write down a list of 10 major goals you would like to achieve in your lifetime.

2) Ask yourself the question, "How many of these goals will I be able to achieve before I die?" Be honest.

3) This number is your CQ. If you <u>really</u>

scored a 10, then please call me so I can

bask in your glow. If you're somewhere

between 3 and 9 like the rest of us, then

keep reading.

There are a number of ways to increase your CQ, but one of the most basic and

productive ways is to "Always Expect Miracles". It sounded silly to me too when I first

heard it, but there is an extremely effective "Method" to what may seem "Madness".

Expecting miracles

Always expecting miracles can only be attained by "Mastering our Expectations." I first

heard of this term while reading the James Redfern book, "The Secret of Shambala". A

wise Tibetan Lama taught the main character in the book to be ever vigilant in

monitoring the expectations he had of himself as well as others. Without mastering this,

the main character was told he would never reach the paradise of Shambala. Making

realistic application of this approach requires three things:

1) Remaining present and conscious of your thoughts.

2) Knowing what your preferred expectations truly are.

3) Having faith in the everyday potential for miracles. Taking a

   moment to feel the electricity in the air. Waiting for "it"

   at the edge of your seat. If you're brave enough, thanking your

   guides & angel(s) for the miracles they're waiting to give you.

My own experience with mastering expectations happened on a car trip from my home in Northern New Jersey to Manhattan. I was on a three lane highway heading east, listening to Redfern's book on tape. The melodious voice of Lavar Burton just finished reading a section on how to:

1) Create a field of loving energy around you.

2) Extend this field out to someone you're focusing on.

3) Increase the vibration of that person's

   energy field until they begin to make

   decisions from a point of love not fear and anger.

The way it was presented, it almost seemed like it could <u>possibly</u> work. Suddenly, this fanciful thought was rudely interrupted by an angry tailgater in a fancy Italian sports car. I was going 65 in a 55 and he was literally three feet behind me. I could see the expression on his face from the rear view mirror, and he wasn't a happy camper. Before I had a chance to react, a strange sense of calmness came over me. I thought, "Before I resort to flipping him the bird, I'm going to try the energy technique I just learned. I've got to believe this guy's a good person who's just a bit stressed." I felt empowered by giving myself a chance to be proactive instead of reactive. I felt a tingle down my spine. Electricity in the moment. Would the potential of a small miracle unfold? I began building my energy field with each deep breath. I visualized sending this loving field out to the driver behind me. In my mind's eye, I saw the vibration of his field elevate. Within a few seconds, he came up to my right side, SMILED at me, and accelerated into the distance. This same exact thing happened three more times on the trip to Manhattan. My drive to NYC turned into an intensive workshop on "Mastering my Expectations" &

"Expecting Miracles". When I finally got to my parking garage on west 43rd street, I wondered if it was all a dream. But no...It was real.

Appreciating & Remembering Miracles

Would my experience turn into a forgotten dream? A miracle not properly filed in gray matter. Would I question it's very existence at a later date? All I knew is I wanted to hold onto this spark, this memory, this feeling. The stresses of the day were coming on fast and the morning's events already seemed months in the past. How could something so wonderful fade away so quickly, only to be replaced with the frustrations of a finite reality. Suddenly, it came to me! I can't possible allow the events of the morning to be forgotten. I ran into the first stationary store I could find, and bought a journal. It was small enough to carry around in my suit pocket so It would always be accessible to record things like this right after they happen. I hurriedly filled in two and a half pages with the events and sensations I had experienced during my commute into the city. Then I made three promises to myself:

1) I would make it a point to record miracles in my book within at most two hours of experiencing them.

2) I would take at least 15 minutes each morning to review this ever evolving list.

3) I would do my best each day to wake up with the following words in my head, "I have witnessed miracles in my life, and I look forward to experiencing more today."

You can't see an angel
if you don't take the time to recognize them

What if witnessing miracles wasn't a matter of waiting around for that rare event; but instead, changing the way you look at the world so you can see miracles happen every moment. What if you truly felt life was a miracle? What would you do, attempt, or experience?

I once asked myself these questions when I was sitting at an outdoor café in lower Manhattan. It was a balmy summer evening. I had just finished eating dinner at an Italian restaurant down the street, and I came to the café to have a cup of Earl Grey Tea. I pulled out a metallic paper weight that I bought from a shop on the upper west side. The question, "What would you attempt if you knew you could not fail?", was engraved on it's surface. I thought to myself, "someone would really have to believe that they were living in a world of miracles to manifest something like this in their life."

I took a few more sips of my tea, and suddenly a sharp image of an old yoga teacher came to mind? I remembered what he told me once about breathing. He said, "In the west people think they're just breathing in gases like oxygen and nitrogen, but in the east we see breath and the air we breathe in as an energetic blessing. In India we call it PRANA." I remembered a breathing technique and visualization he'd taught me several years back. I put down my teacup and began to put that lesson into action. I slowly inhaled through my nose. At the same time I visualized a ground mist of white light begin to enter my body through my feet. As the light entered me I felt a great warmth and security. Almost as if I was being loved unconditionally. When I was filled with the light and my lungs had seemingly reached their capacity, I forced in three more quick puffs of air. I held the breath and saw the light begin to gently over flow out the top of my head like a water fountain. After about ten seconds I started to exhale through my mouth. I chose not to release the misty cloud of light; but instead, a murky grey exhaust that was the essence of my sadness, anger, and fear. It exited through my feet and the earth accepted it freely. For some strange reason, I knew the earth would transmute these energetic emotions into the loving light of Prana, so I released them without guilt or regret. At the point I could exhale no more, I forced out three more puffs of air. After holding my breath for three seconds, I began to inhale through my nose and start the process over again.

After five minutes of this, my mind couldn't hold thoughts of worry or anger. After fifteen minutes my surroundings began to glow as if every object was illuminated from within. After thirty minutes, my level of awareness and sense of abundance were so intense that I had to pay the check and explore the streets of SoHo. I walked down Prince Street with a wide smile on my face as I looked into every shop window I could find. I had walked down this street hundreds of times in the past; but until now I had never noticed the melodious sounds of café music, the enticing scents of culinary herbs and imported espresso, and the beautiful designs, shapes and colors to be found in every boutique window. I took a right onto Broadway. Walked for awhile, then took a left onto Spring Street. Suddenly I was standing in front of a small shop that specialized in Alternative Spirituality, Natural medicine, and anything else that could be labeled esoteric. I walked in and felt like a kid in a candy shop. There were books on everything from Buddhism to natural treatments for back pain, Astrology to Acupuncture, Magic spells to Mountain climbing in Tibet. I was expecting to find a book entitled, "The

True Story of Harry Potter", when everything around me lost it's Vibrant glow.

Everything became monochrome and unappealing. I looked up and saw a book entitled,

"Time to Leave". For some reason I saw this more as a message than a coincidence, so I

left. Just as I hit the sidewalk, I was face to face with a friend that I had been trying to

find for the past 17 years. She was my first true love. We spoke intensely for hours, never

breaking eye contact. As we hugged goodbye, I noticed that everything was glowing

again, and I was left with a tremendous feeling of closure. I walked away with the

knowledge that for a short while I had experienced the ultimate truth. "Persistent focus

and a clear intention to remain present will inevitably reveal the ever present stream of

miracles that guide and nurture us all."

A moment for a pat on the back..

Did you ever ask yourself what part YOU truly play in the creation of miracles, or have

you fully relegated their manifestation to those who inhabit the angelic realms? Would

you be surprised to know that you play just as important a role in the bringing of miracles

as any angel, or even God?

Taking charge at the "Angel Employment Agency"

Those of you who believe there's no such thing as God, Angels, or even an after life, may

not resonate with the information on in the next few paragraphs. If you do believe, or are

open, read on.

I once had a conversation with an intuitive healer about Angels and their intentions. She told me, "In a world of disbelievers, Angels are like Maytag Repairmen. When people don't confirm their existence by asking for their assistance, they simply sit, watch and wait." Unlike some people, Angels don't get the concepts of unemployment and retirement. They exist to serve. In life, we have all the angelic help we could ever need. The challenge for many is to recognize that fact, and be open to receiving it.

Affirmation: Asking like you believe it's going to happen

The simple act of "Asking" for something always includes some amount of doubt that your request will be honored. If you really knew that you were going to get something, you wouldn't ask, but instead, affirm that it was going happen by showing thanks. In the Lord's Prayer we say, "Give us this day our daily bread", not, "Please give us bread!" The former is an affirmation. The later is a request with some degree of disbelief that it will really happen.

So at this point you're probably saying, "I'd like to experience more miracles in my life." But, know this. Miracles are the greatest catalyst for change in a person's life. Be open to miracles, but in the same light, be open to change. If not, your miracles won't be experienced with regularity. This is why I've chosen the daily affirmation, "In my life I have seen many miracles. Thank you for bringing me the miracles I will experience today. I am open to the path of conscious evolution and any changes needed to promote this process."

Celebrating Miracles

The best way to give thanks for miracles is to celebrate their existence. What I'm talking about is not new. In fact, it's as old as celebrating Christmas or Passover; But, in this case you are rejoicing in miracles that you've personally experienced. This transforms the celebration from one of social ceremony to an expression of conscious evolution.

Celebrate with one friend or a dozen. The tone can be serious or comical. It can include anything from meditation to Beatles music. Like my great uncle the band leader used to say, "It's your gig." There are just a few things you may want to remember in creating this event.

- Everyone should have an opportunity to share at least one miracle with the group.
- Remember. It's not a miracle competition. So don't judge or quantify the significance of other miracles.
- Recognizing and experiencing a miracle to further your spiritual evolution is often times more important than the miracle itself.

Chapter 4
**Biology, Psychology
& Spirituality;
The Interdependent Triad**

You are a great work of art that never stops painting itself anew. Shapes, colors, and compositional intent. All moving, growing, evolving. Art that experiences itself and the world around it. The shapes are your physical structure and the things you manifest in your world. Colors are your psyche and emotional disposition. The composition and intent are an expression of your souls direction and purpose. When all the elements of this masterpiece work in harmony, it's message to the world is clear. When these elements compete, or are at odds with each other, problems may arise.

Biology's Effect on Psychology.

There are numerous ways that biochemical imbalances, nutrient insufficiencies, allergies, toxicity, Chronic Pain or infections can adversely affect your emotional state. Here are just a few:

Diet

As a nutritional consultant for a major vitamin supplement provider, I've worked very closely with hundreds of Mainstream and Alternative medical practitioners to help provide solutions to their patient's health issues. In my experience, one of the biggest threats to a healthy psyche is the "American Diet". Problems with dietary intake can be broken into four main categories; Nutrient deficiency and excess, blood sugar imbalance, and food allergies.

1) **Nutrient Deficiency**:

    a) **Protein**: The Amino Acids that make up the proteins we eat are essential in the production neurotransmitters for proper mood and brain function. In a culture filled with snack foods, sweets, soda pop, and novice vegetarians; optimal intake of high quality proteins is often an afterthought. As a general rule, a reasonably healthy individual without kidney problems should consume around 75 grams of high quality protein on a daily basis. A minimum of 15 grams of protein at any meal. Each meal should contain a combination of protein, healthy fats, and complex carbohydrates. For any of you who practice "food combining"; remember, you can get your carbs from vegetables.

    b) **Vitamins & Minerals**: Both the Vitamin B6 and the Mineral Magnesium play an important role in the production of the neurotransmitter "Serotonin". This substance is well known for it's role in the regulation of mood. Increasing your intake of whole grains for Vitamin B6 and dark green leafy vegetables for Magnesium can help to decrease your risk of deficiencies in these two essential nutrients.

Nutrient Excess:

a) **Manganese:** In the later part of the 1900s, mothers with lactose intolerant infants gave their children soy based formulas as an alternative to dairy. A well known Long Island based hospital research center followed these children into adolescence. They noticed an alarming rate of violent criminal behavior in these children as opposed to the ones who were breast feed or had received dairy based formulas. After extensive investigation, these localized the problem to the excessive Manganese content in soy based infant formulas. In fact, these formulas contained <u>hundreds of times</u> the Manganese content found in mothers milk, and dozens of times the Manganese found in simple soy milk. Remember to read the label. Dietary sources of Manganese are best measured in Micrograms (Mcgs), not Milligrams (Mgs).

Blood Sugar Imbalance:

I was only 7 years old when I first experienced the effects a simple biochemical imbalance could have on a person's emotional state. It was a cool, crisp Thanksgiving evening, and my mother ,(God bless her for putting up with us), had just cleared the dirty dishes from the dinning room table. We all gathered in the living room around a roaring fire that my father had lit for the occasion. Mom asked each one of us if we wanted a piece of apple pie ala mode. When she turned to my father she said, "None for you honey. Remember. You don't do well with sweets." Suddenly, his gentle demeanor changed, and he snapped at her with a, "I WANT A PIECE! I'LL BE ALRIGHT!" My mother gave him a dirty look, then hurried off to the kitchen. Moments later, she came back with our dessert, and everyone dug in. The crackling sounds of the fire were nearly drown out by clinking of forks against porcelain and the non stop "MMM MMMM MMM" that came from my father as he inhaled his portion of pie and ice cream. Afterwards, I helped my mom take the dirty dessert plates to the kitchen sink. When I returned to the living room, my father was sitting quietly in his big comfy chair staring at the dancing flames in the fireplace. I said, "Fire's going good dad." But he didn't respond. He didn't even blink. I thought this was strange, so I added, "Dad…Did you hear me?" His face turned to me and his eyes filled with a crazed anger as he yelled, "What the hell are you bothering me for!!!" My mother burst into the room, gave my father another dirty look, then escorted me into the kitchen. She looked down at me and said, "Sometimes sugar makes daddy mean. He's not mad at you. It's just the sugar." When I was a little older my brother told me that dad suffered from Reactive Hypoglycemia (Low Blood Sugar). Unfortunately, every time he ate sweets, he wasn't the only one to suffer.

For those who are sensitive to refined carbohydrates (Sweets), it's important to note that the problem is not necessarily the eating of these foods, but the speed in which the sugar gets absorbed through the intestines and enters the bloodstream. Eating carbs alone, (like a box of cookies), elevates blood sugar rapidly; and your chance of experiencing mood swings will increase. On the other hand, when you combine carbs along with things like protein, healthy fats, or fiber; you slow the absorption of sugar into the bloodstream. This will not only help to stabilize your mood, but also your energy levels. One trick I learned from a savvy nutritionist in Manhattan was to always have "rescue protein" on hand. So the next time you break into the Valentines Day chocolates on a midnight raid of the kitchen, make sure you have some Hard Boiled Eggs, Broiled Chicken Cutlets, or Freshly Sliced Turkey Breast in the fridge to eat afterwards. These proteins will not only help you avoid the "Sugar Blues" by slowing the absorption of sugar into your bloodstream, but reduce your chances of putting on extra fat from your late night indulgence as well.

Food Allergies:

I once took a prominent doctor and his wife out to dinner at a fashionable French restaurant on lower Park Avenue in Manhattan. We had reservations, but we still waited 30 minutes to be seated. We ordered almost immediately, but it took another 45 minutes before we received our appetizers. In the meantime, the waiter dropped off some fresh hot bread and butter to our table. As soon as the bread basket hit the red striped tablecloth, the doctor dove into the bread with almost an addictive fury. With ever bit the doctor took, his wife got more and more upset. I wondered why she reacted so. The doctor was not over weight, so his wife couldn't be concerned about his calorie intake. After about his fourth piece, his wife said sharply, "Enough with the bread!" The doctor's jaws froze mid chew. He quietly put his bread down, quickly chewed and swallowed what he had in his mouth; then turned to me. "So...Adam...tell me about that new natural pain formula your company has been promoting", said the doctor. I pulled a presentation binder out of my case and began the 10 minute process of detailing this product to the doctor. For the first two minutes, he seemed very enthusiastic about the research I was presenting. About three minutes into it, I noticed he was beginning to stare off into the distance and became less and less responsive to the high points of my presentation. I tried to get him back into it with a few questions about his practice, but it almost seemed as if he had gone deaf. He was no longer responding to any of my questions. It was almost like I wasn't even there. I was starting to get a little impatient at this point, so I raised my voice and said, "Doctor!....are you with me on this?" It was almost like I broke him out of a trance as he said, "I'm sorry Adam…I really shouldn't of had that bread." "You know you have problems with wheat. Why do you do this to yourself?", said his wife. We ate the rest of our meal in near silence. I paid the check, said goodbye, and waived them down a cab. I tried to get another appointment with him on numerous occasions without success. A few months later, I was informed by one of his associates that he was still too embarrassed to meet with me.

Chronic Pain

Of all the health concerns that can effect ones state of mind, Chronic pain can be the most daunting. On September 9th, 1990, my wife Robin and I were married. We had a beautiful wedding, but this story starts with the reception. After the meal, our band started to play some great 80s pop music. Everyone was dancing, and a group of husbands and boyfriends got Robin and me to sit in a couple of chairs as they lifted us in the air and paraded us around the dance-floor. All of the sudden, one of the men who was holding me up, tripped, and down I went from a height of seven feet. After hitting the floor, I felt a slight strain in my back, but I had so much champagne in me that I just kept on dancing and socializing. I woke up the next morning to a pain in my back that I will never forget. I got out of bed like a crippled man, but the worst was yet to come. In an hour, Robin and I would be hopping into the car for an eight hour drive to Maine and our honeymoon.

For the first and second days of our trip, I simple kept the pain to myself and whimpered as little as possible. On the third day, I began to loose my patience when confronted with minor inconveniences. By the eighth day, I was loosing my ability to keep focused during conversations. When the last day of our honeymoon rolled around, I was so beaten down by the pain that I became profoundly depressed. Thank god I found a good chiropractor when we returned home to NYC.

It only took 2 weeks of intense chronic pain to turn my world inside out. I can't even imagine experiencing this level of pain for a matter of years, like numerous fibromyalgia patients do. Since then, I've lecturing to various groups of doctors on the subject of "Pain", and here are some of the highlights:

- NSAIDs (Non-Steroidal Anti-inflammatory Drugs) though effective, also have major draw backs as well. They can lead to gastric bleeding in as little as three weeks of continuous use.
- Selective COX-2 Inhibitors like Vioxx and Celebrex were supposed to resolve that issue, but even they can cause gastric bleeding at times.
- Many rheumatologists would agree that low dose steroidal anti-inflammatories

like "Prednisone", would be a better choice for chronic pain.

- Herbs like Turmeric, Ginger, Boswellia, Hops and Rosemary are beginning to show some impressive results in preliminary pain studies.

- Frequency Specific Micro-current devices might prove to be one of the most interesting, low cost and effective ways to treat chronic pain. Do not confuse this with simple micro-current.

- A diet that is low in red meats, sugar, unhealthy fats, alcohol, caffeine; while being high in green leafy veggies & fish, tends to reduce inflammation in your body. This lifestyle modification is aptly know as an "Anti-Inflammatory Diet."

- Free Radicals from environmental pollutants activate something in you body known as NFKappaB, which in turn promotes inflammation. Try to steer clear of household pesticides, breathing in nail polish, and breathing in excessive bus and car exhaust.

- Having too high a percentage of body fat can increase overall levels of inflammation in your body. This can aggravate and enhance chronic pain. Numerous studies published in well respected medical journals have documented this fact. Loosing weight can be a challenge, but keeping it on can be a real pain.

Thyroid Issues

Sub-Optimal thyroid function is a modern day epidemic that effects tens of millions of people each year. When your thyroid is not optimally functioning, you may suffer from symptoms like fatigue, depression, hopelessness, brain fog, weight gain, constipation, and that's just the short list. To understand thyroid issues, it's important to understand both the purpose and function of this important endocrine gland. Your thyroid gland is the gas pedal to increase or decrease the metabolic function of most every organ and structure in your body. For example, if you are hyper thyroid, you may suffer from high blood pressure; conversely hypothyroidism may produce low blood pressure. Hyperthyroid people tend to be thin and burn calories quickly, while those with Hypo-thyroidism may put on weight easily because they store calories as fat, instead of burning them for energy. Hypothyroidism can also contribute to emotional problems due to lowered energy production in brain tissue.

Between 1998 and 2001, I had the great privilege of working with Dr. Raphael Kellman in NYC as his co-host on WEVDs "Alternative Medicine Update". On this weekly radio program we would discuss the prevalence and natural treatment of Thyroid, Adrenal and Gastrointestinal disorders. In preparing research for these shows, I've gained some valuable insights for people suffering from Thyroid issues.

- If you're tired, depressed, gaining weight, losing hair, and have tested negative for thyroid issues using the standard panels (T4 & TSH); then the test may not be picking up your thyroid issue. Go to a practitioner that can administer and properly interpret the "TRH" (Thyroid Response Hormone) test. This test can pick up thyroid problems when normal panels can't.

- Adrenal dysfunction can contribute to thyroid issues. When you get stressed out, your adrenal glands excrete a substance called "Cortisol. Chronic elevated cortisol can inhibit thyroid function & hormone production. This is one of the mechanisms by which stress and depression are connected. There are a number of ways to curb cortisol production after experiencing stress, but the easiest and least costly way is by doing deep breathing exercises within 2 minutes after the exposure to stress. Slowly breathing in thru your nose and out through your mouth can help to reduce many of the side effects of stress. Ten deep breaths can really make a difference, emotionally and bio-chemically.

- Increases in estrogen, via Estrogen Replacement may reduce your thyroid function by lowering the amount of free thyroid hormone in your body. This is another thing to consider when deciding if estrogen replacement is right for you.

Learn to Love your Guts

If the world is a stage, then the cast of characters is nearly 5 billion strong. The same could be said of the microcosm we call the human intestines. Billions of organisms (bacteria, yeasts, parasites, etc), live on the internal landscape of your colon. It would be great if they all got along, but more often than not, it's a battle between the good, the bad, and the indifferent. How you feel physically and emotionally may have a lot to do with who's winning, and who's loosing.

If the population of good bacteria in your intestines is larger than that of the bad bacteria:

-you bloat less after meals,

-your bowel movements are regular,

-you catch colds less frequently, because your immune system is stronger,

-and you just generally feel happier.

If the bad organisms out number the good ones, then you:

-increase your risk of Intestinal bloating and cramping

-may suffer from bowel irregularity (constipation & diarrhea)

-are more susceptible to opportunistic infections & food poisoning

-tend to be less energetic and more emotionally fragile.

If you suffer from Irritable Bowel Syndrome, Colitis, Inflammatory Bowel Disease, or any of the symptoms listed above; you may want to try a well researched intestinal cleansing protocol known as the "4R Program". This approach to promote intestinal health was created and studied by Dr. Jeffrey Bland and his associates at the Functional Medicine Research Center in Gigg Harbor, Washington. Teaching this approach to healthcare providers in NYC has yielded such phenomenal patient outcomes, that I would be remise if I did not share it with you.

Each of the "4R"s is a Phase of the program. The first "R" is for Remove. In this phase we remove foods that the patient may be intestinally sensitive to, like wheat & dairy. You also want to remove any pathogenic organisms, like unfriendly bacteria, yeasts, or parasites. There are numerous pharmaceutical agents that can effectively remove these organisms, but many have unpleasant side effects like stomach upset and diarrhea. Certain natural therapeutics can do the job without the side effects.

They are:

- Berberine Sulfate: from berberine containing herbs like oregon grape, has been studied for it antimicrobial characteristics.

- Artemisia annua: or wormwood, has been used to kill parasites by indigenous culture for hundreds of years. It's safe and effective when properly dosed.
- Red Thyme Oil: is rich in the active substance "Thymol". It's ability to control the growth of unfriendly yeast is impressive.

The Second "R" is for Restore. In this phase we need to promote the production of digestive enzymes, and if needed, stomach acid. Stomach acid is one of the most misunderstood substances in western civilization. If you were to believe the multi billion dollar drug companies that produce anti-acids and acid blockers, any time you have the slightest digestive upset, it's due to the enemy; "Stomach Acid!" Unfortunately, this is the furthest thing from the truth. Most stomach upset is actually due to LOW stomach acidity, not high. To prove this, I invite you to try an experiment. The next time your stomach feels bloated and achy after a meal, instead of taking an anti-acid, try a teaspoon of Agostura Bitters. You'll notice your stomach will soon stop bloating and the achyness will go away. This flies in the face of the "Bad Acid" model because the main ingredient in these bitters is Gentiana Lutea. This herb is well known for it's ability to increase your stomachs production of HCL (stomach acid). Having high enough levels of stomach acid also works to kill bad bacteria, like E.Coli, before it can enter into you intestines and make you sick. People with low stomach acidity are much more suceptable to food poisoning than people with normal HCL production. Lastly, people with low stomach acidity tend to have more lower bowel gas and food allergies.

According to the clinical findings of the practitioners I've worked with, a combination formula of HCL, Pepsin, & Gentiana Lutea is the best supplement for low stomach acidity. Please note: if you have a history of, or have been diagnosed with and ulcer, you should not be taking an HCL supplement.

Digestive enzymes like amylase, protease, and lipase are mostly produced by the pancreas, and are dumped into the small intestines to help you digest carbohydrates, proteins, and fats (respectively). In a response to low stomach acid production, your pancreas produces less of these enzymes. When you have inadequate amounts of these enzymes, your food can not be properly digested, and you may not be digesting, absorbing, and utilizing enough nutrients from you food. This may lead to reduced organ function and the onset of fatigue and certain forms of depression.

Finding a high quality digestive enzyme that will be potent enough to do the job, can be tricky. Here are a few important guidelines when choosing the right one.

1) Read the label. Always make sure the enzymes are measured in units of activity (like "USP"s), not by weight (like Mgs or Mcgs). You could have an entire cup of digestive enzymes, but if they're not active, they're useless.

2) Try not to purchase a formula that mixes HCL with enzymes. Many digestive enzymes are pH sensitive, and this combination will destroy them.

3) Contact the manufacturer, and have them send you a copy of an independent laboratory assay on the potency of the lot number that

your bottle came from. The supplement industry that is not properly governed by the FDA, and this is the only way to assure potency.

The third "R" is for Reinoculate. In this phase we implant friendly bacteria into the small and large intestines. The most researched of these organisms are L. Acidophilus & Bifidobacteria. These forms of bacteria have been shown to:

- Produce substances that inhibit bad bacteria and yeast.
- Have a slight cholesterol lowering effect.
- Reduce the risk to colon cancer.
- Improve bowel regularity
- Improve gastrointestinal immune response (IgA)
- Be helpful for people suffering from Irritable bowel
- Help produce B vitamins from food. Certain B's are needed to produce serotonin (the happiness hormone).

You were originally given these organisms by your mother when you passed through her uterus as she was giving birth to you. If you were delivered with a "C Section", you may not have received that original implantation of good bacteria, and this may have played a factor in your:

- Being a "colicy" baby.
- Developing "Thrush" as an infant.
- Having food sensitivities and/or allergies

- Developing frequent ear infections during childhood
- Childhood and/or adult constipation.

Also, long-term antibiotic use, (over 10 days), can reduce your population of good bacteria. Reinoculation with friendly bacteria would also be beneficial for people in this situation as well.

The last "R" is repair. In this phase you'll work to heal the wall of the small and large intestines. When the wall of the intestines is healthy it's "Selectively Permeable". This means it lets some things get through to the bloodstream, (like nutrients), and keeps other things out, (like toxins and undigested matter). When unfriendly bacteria begin to predominate in the intestines, they produce by-products that eventually breakdown the selective permeability of the wall. When undesirable substances, like toxins and undigested proteins are able to enter the bloodstream, they are quickly identified and attacked by cells of your immune system. Often, these same immune cells will then become confused and attack native tissues in your body. This process has been coined "Molecular Mimicry" by the researchers, and has begun to be seen as the cause of many Auto-Immune Disorders like Rheumatoid Arthritis. Healing the wall of the intestines is like sealing the deal for intestinal health. Glutamine, Aloe, and DGL (Licorice), are natural substances that, when combined, are very effective for this.

Remember. If you don't love your own guts, no one else will. Treat them right, and you'll have the intestinal fortitude to stay happy and healthy for a long time to come.

Chapter 5
**Silencing the Panel
of Blind, Negative &
Paranoid Idiots in
your Head**

Something happened. You made an unfortunate decision. Before someone else can come down on you, an automatic mechanism kicks into place, and you come down on yourself. Let me introduce you to the panel of blind, negative and paranoid idiots that live in your head and keep you from realizing your dreams by throwing mud on your self image. Better yet. Let me introduce you to the ones who used to inhabit my head.

Revealing Mine

In an effort to better understand my own self limiting patterns, I decided to give names to these inner gremlins.

The first one I called "Mac", short for Machiavelli. He's the panel member who believes that I'm not willing to do what ever it takes to get the job done. He describes me with words like "Lazy" and "Uncommitted".

The second one who comes to mind would have to be named "Ken", after a young and very idealistic bus boy I worked with when I was a waiter in college. On breaks, Ken and

I used to talk about what we were going to do when we graduated. Unfortunately our conversations would always end in ken calling me a person of "Questionable Intentions." As a matter of fact, Ken was always questioning the integrity of everyone's intentions. I have a leaking suspicion he questioned his own most of all. Ken, the panel member, works relentlessly to make me second guess the integrity of my intentions and the actions I took when interacting with others.

Next would be "Rich". He's the guy I went to college with who became a multi millionaire in corporate marketing. He made it, while I struggled. We were friends once, but he barely acknowledges my existence when I pass him on the street these days. Rich, the panel member, works diligently to encourage my paranoia about being "left behind" or "left out".

Last, but not least is "Sammy". When I first entered high school in Newburgh New York, the coolest kid in 10th grade was "Sammy". Sammy Laforte was the Captain of the soccer team. He was so physically fit, he could do a back flip from a stand still position, without even using his hands. His popularity transcended the barriers of group titles like, "Motorheads, Jocks, and Stoners." The coolest kids in every group were his best friends. If you were his friend, you were "cool". Sammy and I didn't get along to well, so I was considered "Uncool", and Sammy was always the first one to remind me that I just didn't fit in with him and his friends. Sammy, the panel member, finds great joy in reminding me that I don't fit in with the cool crowd on a social basis.

The Panel in Action:

It was a cool and cloudy Sunday morning in April, and my family and I were driving to upstate New York to visit an old friend of my wife who she hadn't seen for a number of years.

As we made the final turn on the directions to her house, we saw it in the distance. It was a quarter mile away and up on a hill. It seemed large from this distance, and when we rolled up it's private driveway lined with perfectly manicured hedges, we realized it was a full-blown mansion. Robin had told me that John, (her friend Marion's husband), was a senior executive at a major advertising agency, but I never thought they were doing this well. We drove around the house to a large private parking lot in back behind their pool & tennis court. We walked back to the front door, and rang the bell. After about 2 minutes the door opened, and there stood John, Marion and their three little boys, all perfectly dressed in the latest L.L.Bean casual wear. I could of sworn that I saw this same family portrait in the latest issue of "Success" magazine. John reached out his hand to mine, shook it, introduced himself and his family, then invited us to a so called "little get together" in the parlor room. When we got there, Robin and I realized that John's idea of a "little get together" was a catered party for fifty being entertained by a classical pianist. All of the sudden my two boys were being dragged off to play with their children, and Robin ran off with her friend Marion. I was left all alone to make small talk with John and the Captains of Industry.

After a glass of white wine and a few pieces of sushi, John came over and asked me to join him and his friends over by the grand piano. When I came over, John introduced me, and said I was in "Healthcare". This got a few nods of approval from the group, then the distinguished looking man with the salt and pepper hair who was standing to the left of John said, "Hey, since we have some new people here, why don't we play STOCK TIP?" Most of them nodded their heads, and John started first. After telling the group about a promising new company that was going IPO in the fall, John passed the ball to the next man. Each person shared there own insights and secrets about stocks and bonds, until it came time for me to talk.John said, "Now it's Adam's turn. Adam, your in healthcare. Are there any hot opportunities in Biotech you know about?"

"Not really", I responded.

"Then where do <u>you</u> put your money these days?" said John

"Well…after a few home improvements, bills, taxes and a yearly contribution to my IRA, I'm pretty tapped out. "

After saying that, I looked up and saw that all the members of John's group were staring at me with puzzled looks on their faces.

The following moments of deafening silence were like an open invitation for the panel of gremlins in my head to voice their opinions. It went something like this:

<u>Rich</u>: "What's a matter Adam? Forgot where you were? Like, way over your head. The difference between these guys and you is that they've made their marks on the blackboard of life, and you forgot to pickup the chalk."

<u>Mac</u>: "99% Perspiration and 1% Inspiration. These guys live by the rules of success. I haven't seen you sweat a drop, except for when John asked you what <u>YOU</u> do with your money."

<u>Ken</u>: "These guys with their over priced polo shirts and khakis. They look squeaky clean, but check what's jammed between the treads on the undersides of their tennis shoes. That's right. The blood and guts of people like you and me. The people they choose to step on so they could make it to this party. .... But you probably envy them don't you. You suck just as much as they do!"

Sammy: "Hey Kenny boy. You can shut it now, or I can shut it for you. These guys are alright by me. But on the other hand, you and Adam would have to reach pretty high just to make it to the bottom of <u>their</u> shoes!"

Suddenly the word, "Honey!" blurted out of my mouth, "I think I heard my wife.....excuse me." I bolted from the hot-seat and went out on the patio to search for my wife and kids in the English Garden behind the estate. Thankfully, Robin and the boys had a good time, so we headed out and arrived back home just a few hours later.

Giving them a job review.

After identifying and describing each one of these characters, I recognized that they were all "State of Mind Consultants" that I never consciously hired. They just sort of moved in and took their positions on the panel when I wasn't looking. But, since I'm the boss here, I get to choose who stays and who goes. So, as a good manager of my thoughts and anything that might influence them, I decided to give each one of these guys a "Job Review."

So there I am, sitting in a large leather chair, behind an impressive birds eye maple desk, in a large corner office with a view of the city. I reach for the intercom on my desk and press a button. "Nancy.. Could you send in the first Idiot?.....I mean panel member...... Thank You." In walks a short and slight man in his late thirties. His hair is conservatively short, dusty blond and parted to the side. His eyes are small and his nose is proportionately too large for his face.

"Rich" I say, "Welcome....come on in and have a seat." He looks around and the only other seat in the room is a short and very uncomfortable looking wooden stool. Rich looks at it in disgust and says, "You expect ME to......."

"YES" I interrupted, "or you can get out......for good!"

"Alright, I'll sit", he said, "but only because I just couldn't bear not being able to kick you when you're down." I smiled, pulled a pen and pad from the desk draw, and began writing. "Hey! ... What's with the note taking?" he said. I looked up from the note paper, smiled and said, "It has come to my attention that certain consultants in my "State of Mind Division" have been working to sabotage a number of core company initiatives. According to recent records from our internal affairs department, you and a number of other consultants have been responsible for the recent "John & Marion's Mansion" incident. This type of public humiliation to Adam Banning Unlimited can not, and **will not** be tolerated!"

"Adam...What are you going to do?...Fire ME!?", interrupted Rich.

"No" I replied, "I'm going to do better than that.....I'm going to replace you!"

With those words, a bolt of lightening came flying through the open window, and hit

Rich in the hollow part of his chest. The same part where most other people keep their hearts. In an instant he was transformed into a much older man with kinder eyes. He sort of looked like my favorite grandfather who my siblings and l always addressed fondly as "Syd". I smiled cautiously and said, "Hello....Good to have you on board. Are you familiar with our company's mission statement. If you like, I can have one of our staffers bring a copy to your new office down the hall." He calmly smiled and replied, " Thanks, but that won't be necessary. I know all about you Adam, and that's why I volunteered for the position. You're a mench (Jewish for a man with integrity) and I won't steer ya' wrong.....Promise."

"Thanks", I said as I giggled slightly. He got up and started towards the door when I added, "Do you mind if I call you Syd?"

"Always worked for me", he replied and then walked out.

All of the other staff changes went about the same way except for Sammy who tried to take a swipe at me, so I had to call security. These days, with my new panel of consultants, negative self talk just doesn't have a chance at Adam Banning Unlimited.

Chapter 6
**See Yourself
Through the
Eyes of Others
to Recognize
the Giant Within**

How would you describe yourself? What are your strengths & weaknesses? Do you think it would be the same as what your friends, associates, and loved ones would say about you? Who would be right? You or them?

It was a beautiful September morning in 2002, but I only got brief glimpses of the breathtaking foliage from the podium I was lecturing from. I was in an over air conditioned hotel lecture room teaching a group of doctors about a naturopathic approach to treating fatigue. I really enjoyed the subject so I gave an enthusiastic presentation. I rapped up at about 1pm, and the doctor's and I headed down stairs to the restaurant for lunch. I was famished. I excused myself from the others and took a table by myself because I had to prepare to give another seminar on Gastrointestinal health that evening. After finishing my food, I heard my name being mentioned in the distance. Two tables away, some of the doctors who attended my presentation were sharing their thoughts about it. I usually try not to listen in on other peoples conversations, but I was wondering what this specific group of influential doctors thought of my presentation. Instead of talking about the content of my seminar, they focused on ME. My presentation skills and knowledge base to be specific. This group of renowned physicians and published authors were using words like, "Brilliant", "Charismatic" and "Paradigm Shifting" to describe me and a presentation that I would rate as a little better than average. I was shocked. I mean I really like lecturing, but I never thought of myself as "Charismatic", never mind "Brilliant"!

Later that night many thoughts ran through my mind. "Am I too close to myself to see who I really am?" "How would my life be different if I truly saw myself as "Brilliant" & "Charismatic?" This reminded me of a saying that I got from a popular motivational speaker. "You will fulfill the destiny of the person you believe you are." Lastly, "If I've been consistently underestimating myself, then where do I go to find a more precise picture of Adam Banning?"

Collecting the Views of Others

The real questions were "Who knew me best?" and "What would be the best way to gather this info from this select group of family, friends, and associates?" So, I created a simple form that had a single question at the top of it, "If you were to use 10 descriptive words to tell someone else about Adam Banning, what would they be?" I then picked ten people to give the forms to along with self addressed stamped envelopes. I instructed each of these people to:

- answer the question honestly,
- not to put their names on the forms or on the return address of the envelopes I provided them,
- Finish them and send them back as soon as possible.

I waited until I received all of the questionnaires back before I began opening them. I tell ya, if you ever needed a royal ego boost, try doing this sometime. I mean it wasn't all good news, but for the most part I was looking at least 50% better than I've ever viewed myself.

Well, this was great for me, but I wondered what would happen if other people tried this with their friends and loved ones. After asking 7 people, 4 decided to do it, and the 3 that got back to me with their responses had similar outcomes to my own. Not only did all 4 of us receive grades substantially higher than we would have given ourselves, but we were also told we had characteristics that we weren't previously aware of. I can still remember the look on my friend Alex's face as he read his questionnaires. He smiled and blushed like he just got the Academy Award for "Best Person on Earth". After reading 3 or 4 of them, he stared out into the distance with a confused look on his face, and asked, "Do you think I'm Inspirational? Two of them thought I was INSPIRATIONAL?!" I always thought he was, but I guess I never told him.

Recognizing the Angel in the Mirror: The "50% Rule"

It was nice to see I wasn't alone in this "underestimation of self", but if I was trying to call this a statistically significant study with only 4 people, I was fooling myself. On top of that, I had a very strong suspicion that there were some sub-groups of people that wouldn't get the same responses as the 4 of us got.

After getting responses back from 32 more people, (making it a total of 36), the score was 24 who "Underestimated" and 12 who either "Properly Estimated" or "Over Estimated" themselves when compared to the views of others. So my next question to answer was, "What differentiated the 24 "under-estimators" from the other 12?" After hitting the internet , five psychology textbooks, and a few journals of Psychiatry; I came up with a theory on how a person could differentiate which group they'd be a member of.

I proceeded to call up each of the 35 participants and compliment them for having the positive traits that their friends and loved ones used to describe them with. There were three different types of responses to these compliments which precisely matched the following three groups of people:

- **"Over-Estimators"**- consistently responded with "Okay" or "Alright" as if it were a confirmation of what they already knew.

- **"Proper-Estimators"**- Always gave a sincere "Thank You", and a few of them thanked me for recognizing those traits in them. By the way, this group of 5 participants were amongst the most successful and accomplished in the whole group of 36.

- **"Under-Estimators"**- (which included me)- seemed uncomfortable receiving compliments and would never just say "Thank You". Their responses were more like modest denials of each compliment.

For a number of months after this experiment I made it a point of observing how people react to compliments. I spent days in a row just complimenting dozens of friends, loved ones, clients and even strangers. This confirmed my previous findings that the majority of people fall into the "Under-Estimators" category.

At this point I was pretty sure that the majority of people were for some reason or another Under Estimators of their own self worth. Using this technique of information gathering was a great short term boost to ones ego, but it lacked lasting effects on creating a positive self image. Basically, you could compliment a person to death, but that doesn't mean their going to believe it, internalize it, and begin acting as if it's true. What to do?..... What to do?...... Eureka! I've got an idea.

Creating the Character

How would my life be different if I accepted and applied all of the talents that others saw in me? How would I handle life's challenges, relationships or my career choices. Could I just snap my fingers, and become this greater me? Probably not, but I could do the next best thing. I could create my own, "Better Self Consultant". Haven't you ever asked yourself "What would so-in-so do in this situation?" Whether it was your supervisor, Superman, or Jesus, it makes no difference. You were taking a person with certain talents and characteristics, and predicting how they would handle a challenge. What if I created a character with all of the positive attributes that I supposedly had, and predicted how that person would go about meeting the same challenges I face in my life? Neat eh? Well here's the character.

His name is Jeffrey Tyler. He is extremely smart, kind, generous, diplomatic, decisive, bold, intuitive to the point of magical, focused, inspiring, a great counselor, teacher, healer, and part time angel. He's a patient and insightful problem solver who can build or fix anything. He's very quick witted, loves animals, and is great with kids. He's empathetic, loyal, and will do almost anything to help a friend in need. He loves a challenge, and is looking forward to helping me with mine. He looks at me with his penetrating green eyes and says, "How may I be of service?"

Asking your consultant for answers: take them for a test run

Well gee…I've got a few challenges in my life. Where should I start? Okay, here's one. I'm having a lot of trouble with keeping my wife from yelling at the kids and me first thing in the morning. Almost every morning she finds things that are bothering her around the house, and her aggravation is only compounded by the stress of getting herself and the kids off in the morning. When she starts to yell, the only thing I can think of is getting out of the house as soon as possible. In my mad run to vacate the premises, I end up forgetting to bring important Items to work like my wallet, cell phone, and day planner. One day I flew out the house so fast that I forgot to bring my son to day camp before heading into New York City for work. That wouldn't have been such a problem if I just left him home; but instead, I forgot he was in the back seat of my car.Unfortunately, I didn't discover that until I was on the New York Side of the George Washington Bridge. He thought it was hilarious, but I didn't get to work until 11am that day, and missed two very important appointments.

"So Jeffrey, how would you handle this one if you were me?" Jeffrey Tyler put both of his hands together. Palm to palm. Finger tips to finger tips. Then he slowly lifted them to his face, with his forefingers to his lips and his thumbs under his chin. He sat there in contemplation for what seemed an eternity, but I was impatient for an answer, so it was probably only a little over a minute. Then he spoke. "If you want your partner to "act" responsibly as opposed to "react" irresponsibly, you must do four things.

 First, claim responsibility for the part you play in her reactivity. Then fess up to her about it with the appropriate apologies.

Second, help to reduce the number and intensity of stressors that trigger her vocalizations of anger and frustration.

Third, communicate a family mission of "Calm Morning Exodus" to your children, and get them to buy in for the sake of a harmonious household environment. Also, inform them of the important role they play in keeping the peace.

Lastly, inform your wife of the benefits and responsibilities of a team member in the consistent pursuit of this family mission.

But Adam, before you "forcibly" implement this program with your family like a bull in a china shop, please keep three things in mind:

1) Communication is not what you say (or even intend to say), but what others hear. There's a big difference, so be mindful and diplomatic with your words.

2) <u>Try</u> not to single out an individual and lay blame upon them, especially in front of others, So, instead of saying "You did it" or "It's your fault", Try "As a family, I think we could do a better job at......." Focusing on "The Family" as opposed to "a family

member", and "Opportunities for Improvement" instead of "Allocating Blame"; sets the stage for new beginnings.

3) After sharing your thoughts with other family members, always ask them, "So, what do you think about that?" It's VERY IMPORTANT to give them an opportunity to express their views on the matter. Remember, listen intently, and show them the respect they deserve as an important member of the team. If you hear them start playing the "Blame Game", let them finish what their saying and gently refocus them on "Team", "Family" and "Opportunities for Improvement".

"So Adam, How does that sound to you?" "GREAT" I replied, "Now let me work on implementation."

That evening I had separate talks with my wife and kids. I confessed my shortcomings, shared my thoughts, and heard theirs without interrupting. The next morning, I woke up an hour earlier than usual to help my wife with her morning chores so she could have at least 15 minutes to sit, relax, and eat her breakfast. This seemed to put her in a great mood, and when my kids got up, they were very calm and helpful as well. I'm crossing my fingers when I say this, but, mornings at the Banning household have been calm with few exceptions ever since. Thank you, Jeffrey Tyler!

I called upon my "Better Self Consultant" for help with a few more challenges in my life. Every time I followed through on his recommendations, my challenges were almost miraculously transformed into opportunities for growth.

Jeffrey Tyler is brilliant! Hold on a second......Jeffrey Tyler is ME??!!! He has all of MY characteristics & abilities. So if I could internalize that fact, I should be able to meet most any challenge in life, and come out on top, Right??? Right??

No! It can't be that easy! Something's missing from this equation. Alright. Let's approach this from the opposite direction. Instead of accepting and promoting the positives, let's identify what things keep me from being Jeffrey Tyler. So I asked myself 2 questions:

First,

Question: What things make me act foolishly, irresponsibly, blindly, or unconsciously?
Answer: Stress & Confrontation. When I get stressed out or I feel like I'm being attacked I say and do some of the most "Anti-Jeffrey Tyler" things you can imagine. So the first block to realizing my true greatness is "Reactivity".

Second,

Question: What else makes me act like someone other than my true self?
Answer: Being a chameleon, and changing the way I present myself to adapt to the needs of the situation. How can I reap the benefits of being me, if "Me" changes every time my environment does. Some people may argue this point by saying, "Adapting to your environment is an essential Survival Skill", but in my experience "Chronic Adaptation"

reduces the amount of time you have to experience the wonders of being "You". In other words, "You can't master Indy Race Car driving by spending more time behind the wheels of SUVs, Minivans, and Tractors.

Chapter Seven
Reactivity and Chronic Adaptation:
The barriers between "who I'm being"
and "the being I am."

Reactivity. Everyone suffers from it to one extent or another. We're the most reactive about our own "Perceived Shortcomings", and everyone has at least a couple of those. As a kid, I thought I was never smart enough in the shadow of my brother's Mega IQ, and never cool enough to possibly be related to my sister, the coolest girl in school.

When I was 12 years old, my father and I spent the day at a ski lodge in the Pocono Mountains of Pennsylvania. My father went there on business, so I had to entertain myself for the day. I didn't like the idea of sliding uncontrollably down a snow covered mountain, even though they called it the, "Bunny Slope", and my father was willing to pay for lessons. Instead, I stayed warm sitting around the roaring circular fire located in the center of the huge chalet. As I was staring into the burning embers, I heard the conversation of two young men in their late teens. "You're going to loose your Queen that way", said the taller of the two. As I looked over, I noticed that they were playing my favorite game, Chess. I got up, and went over to them. I cautiously interrupted, "Do you mind if I watch?" The shorter one with the kind face looked up at me, smiled, and said, "Sure. Have a seat. Maybe you'll learn something." "Not from him, you won't. I'm gonna destroy him." Said the taller blond teen with a cruel snicker. I watched them play for a couple of minutes, then said, "I've got winner." The tall one gave me long gaze of

contempt, and then finally nodded. Over the next 20 minutes, both players gave up a

number of different pieces to each other. Then finally the tall blonde teen took a deep

gratifying breath, moved his black bishop, and proclaimed, "CHECKMATE!" The

shorter teen slumped back into his chair with a look of amazement on his smiling face.

After a moment they were both on their feet, shaking hands and thanking each other for a

good game. The loser left, as the winner sat back down and began to set up the pieces to

play again. I hopped into the now vacant seat and said, "Winners choice. What do you

want, Black or White?" He totally ignored me, stood up looked around the room and

yelled, "Anybody want to play?!" I felt a rage rise from my stomach to my head. The

skin on my face was blazing with heat as I stood up and said, "Hey! I called winner!" He

laughed and said, "I don't play beginners!" "What are you brain-dead! I called winner,

and you nodded yes!", I replied. All of the sudden, he snapped and started yelling curse

words at me until everyone in the busy ski chalet stopped what they were doing and took

notice. When his diatribe of swear words seemed to run dry I screamed, "SCREW YOU,

YOU BASTARD PEICE OF SHIT!" He hauled off and punched me in the chest. It

knocked the wind out of me as I fell backwards onto the cold marble floor. A tall man

about my father's age grabbed the teen as I ran out the door into the cold. I stood in the

cold leaning up against my father's car as I tried to shake off the embarrassment, anger

and pain. About an hour later, my father showed up and we went back home.

Q: How did the spectators version of chess turn into a public swearing match, and finally, assault on a minor?

A: We both had the same insecurities about our intelligence. When he totally ignored me and assumed I was a beginner I became reactive. When I called him brain-dead, he became reactive. When I swore at him and embarrassed him publicly, he became violently reactive. Insecurity breeds unconscious reactivity, which in turn brings out the worst in all parties involved. The proactive spirit of Jeffrey Tyler can only be expressed by those who are willing to identify their insecurities, be conscious of them when they arise, and finally stare them down until they no longer exist. There are two different types of insecurities. Ones that are based in reality, and ones that aren't. For the ones that are based in realty you may want to try the following technique to identify, be conscious of, and overcome them.

1) Get a piece of paper and write down 5 abilities and/or characteristics that you would like to improve upon or acquire. These should be ones that have affected your life negatively by not having or mastering them. If you're being honest with yourself about this list, they may be hot spots of insecurity as well.

2) Have a close friend or relative ask you why you haven't taken the steps to overcome these deficiencies in your life. For the purpose of this technique, you would want to feel as if you've been put on the defensive.

3) As this person interrogates you on each of these 5 items you should begin to notice how and where each subject effects your body and mind. Write down the information. For example:

> **Subject:** My inability to spend wisely and save money.
>
> **Location & Feeling**: Pressure in my chest and lump in my throat.
>
> **Emotion**: Hopelessness

4) Pick the subject you got the most intense physical and emotional response from. Read your notes on the experience and begin to feel it again. The moment your mind and body are back in that space, start to visualize a big red blinking stoplight in front of you. Make it part of the experience. As you focus on the red light, you notice the words "Breathe" & "Feet" in black on the blinking bulb. This will remind you to breath in through your nose and out through your mouth while you concentrate on the souls of your feet. The calming and grounding effect that this will produce can be helpful in diffusing the onset of a reactive state.

Chronic Adaptation:

Did you ever notice that some people act differently around you than they act around other people? If they're the same person, then why don't they act the same around everyone? The concept makes sense, but more often than not it doesn't work out that way. People are social creatures, and like chameleons, being able to adapt to your surroundings is a characteristic considered valuable in today's Western Society. The real question I'd like you to think about is "when does adaptation become so unconscious and frequent that it hinders your own self expression and actualization?"

There are many levels of Chronic Adaptation. Amongst the mildest is a strange but common habit my father had. He would start speaking to someone who had a foreign accent, and begin to take on the accent himself. I'm certain this was his own unconscious attempt to better communicate with the other person, but if you ever had the opportunity to speak with him after he's spent 30 minutes with Japanese clients, you'd swear he just came of the set of a bad Godzilla movie. A habit like this is little more than an annoyance, and probably not going to put too much of a crimp in your self actualization process; but there are number of other unconscious adaptation habits that can.

The Two Main Types of Chronic Adaptation

The "Fit In"

When we were younger they called it "giving into peer pressure". These days we label it as "Not Rocking the Boat", and justify our self imposed uniformity by believing it makes us a productive cog in the machine we call "Society". Let's face it, In some way or another everyone of us tries to "fit in" at one time or another. What other option is there? In today's busy work and social environments, being different from everyone else will more than likely provide you with one or more of three distinct outcomes.

- You become a Leader, Trend Setter, or possibly a "Role Model"
- You could be attacked or persecuted for your views and actions.
- You may just be ignored.

Most people who are willing to share and act upon their unique views don't end up with the first outcome because, as Nelson Mandela once said, "People are not as afraid of their weaknesses as they are of their strengths." To attain the first outcome, one would have to not only understand, but embrace their strengths. This is rare, and probably why Leaders, Trend Setters, and Role Models account for much less than 1% of the world's population. If you don't <u>currently</u> qualify for entrance into that clubhouse, don't worry, read on, be patient in the application of the techniques discussed. Soon you'll be building your own clubhouse, and those folks will be banging at YOUR door to join.

The "Masquerader"

It was a warm, humid and raining day in midtown Manhattan. I had just left my last appointment of the day, and I had an hour to kill before I was meeting a friend for dinner down in Little Italy. I was on the North West Corner of 42nd Street and Fifth Avenue when I looked up and noticed that I was standing in front of Nat Sherman's, one of New York's most famous Cigar Shops. I peaked in the window and noticed they had my favorite cigar in stock. Smoking cigars is not something I do more than a few times a year, but when I do, I smoke those cigars. "This must be an omen!" I walked in, bought the cigar, and headed up to the smoking lounge on the second floor of the store. The lounge was filled with smoke and the sounds of Yankee fans cheering and screaming at a 60 inch flat screen TV on the wall. All of the lounge chairs were taken, so I pulled up a folding chair, lit up my cigar, and began to watch the game. Everyone blasted out with a large shout when Derek Jeter hit the ball for a home run. They all started making comments about Jetter, then Sammy Sosa, then this player, then that player. I started feeling a little out of place, because I knew very little about baseball. Suddenly, one of the older guys in the room brought up Babe Ruth's famous Curse against the Boston Red Socks. Luckily, I watched a piece on the History channel the night before on just that subject. I chimed in, and before you know it, everyone was asking ME my opinion about all the players they loved and hated. With just a tiny bit of knowledge, I became an expert in their eyes, and was excepted into their "Inner Circle".

I fit in, but I felt funny about masquerading as a "Baseball Expert", so I called up my dad. He really WAS a baseball expert. When I told him what happened, and how I felt like a phony, he replied, "I've been in hundreds of smoke filled rooms watching hundreds of games with thousands of guys in my time, and the one thing I've learned for sure is that everyone wants to look like the expert, but no one really is. Everybody in that room was doing the same thing as you were to some degree or another. Don't worry about it kid. It's just another part of male bonding."

My father's words revealed one of the most important reasons why the "Masquerader" in each of us comes to life. Ones level of self-worth is too closely tied to ones level of expertise on any given subject at any given moment. God! How painful and embarrassing can it really be to say, "I really don't know anything about that, but I always wanted to." What if..........?

I woke up early the next morning. Headed down to our neighborhood Starbucks, and sat inside on a big comfy chair with a cup of coffee. A well dressed couple in their 30's sat in the two chairs next to me. They began to converse with each other about their parents, then their children, then the conversation seemed to totally change channels, and they began dissecting the pros and con's of their 401K retirement plans. The woman spoke under her breathe to her husband, as if she were embarrassed to admit something.

He laughed and said, "Everyone with a 401K knows you don't put 90% into high yield, and only 10% into low yield! You'll get killed! Everyone knows that. Here, I'll show you." Then he turns to me and asks, "Do you have a 401K?"

"Yes", I responded.

"Let me ask you a question" he said, "What's your ratio between High Yield High Risk and Low Yield Low Risk investments? I bet Ya it's sure as heck not 90/10!"

I paused and thought, "Help! I really don't know anything about my 401K. My father-in-law the accountant handles all that stuff! This could be embarrassing!.......But, how embarrassing could it really be? This might just be an opportunity!"

After what seemed an eternity, I responded. "To be quite honest, I know next to nothing about my 401k, but I wish I did." A smile came over his face as if he found my honesty refreshing. Then he asked, "Maybe I can help. What would you like to know?"

We spoke for awhile. I asked a lot of questions, and he gave me some advice. I took action on some of his recommendations, and I'm very happy to report that the yield on my 401K has never been better.

In the coming weeks, I had about a dozen more of these "I don't know, but I'd love to learn" type conversations. To my surprise, none of the people I spoke to made me feel dumb for being ignorant about the subjects we discussed. Instead, they seemed to take a certain satisfaction in assuming the role of "teacher" when I eagerly presented myself as their "student".

From that point on I've taken on a new mantra, "I know nothing, but I'd love to learn!" I learned new things about subjects I thought I'd already mastered, subjects I knew nothing about, and subjects I never even knew existed. With this mindset, my thirst for knowledge has doubled and tripled. I feel like a kid again asking, "Why is the sky blue?" for the first time. The world became a bigger place with great new opportunities.

May you always be blessed with a willingness to "accept your ignorance" and the "Curiosity to overcome it". Masquerading that you have knowledge deprives you of your true destiny by limiting the knowledge you can receive and stealing the time you could have spent experiencing your true proactive self. Your own "Jeffrey Tyler".

Discover who you are.

Create who you will be.

But remember, discovering who you are is a process, (or journey), and constantly mirroring others threatens to take you off the path towards your divine destiny.

Chapter Eight
Creative Expression &
the Permanent Smile

Having an outlet for creative expression has really helped me to stay focused,

productive and consciously present. Whether it's writing, journaling, painting,

photography, cooking, or even interior design; having a creative outlet can really help

bring out the best in you. For the past 6 years I've been writing short pieces using

a technique I've coined "Universal Consciousness Poetry".

It all started back in the summer of 1996. It was about 10pm on a Sunday evening, and I

was on the second floor of a Starbucks located on the upper East side of Manhattan. The

crowd cleared out about an hour before, and I was left alone with my laptop and a cup of

Earl Grey tea. I finished the project I was writing for a client, put down the computer, and

began staring out the second story window. Earlier that day I had read an article on the

concept of "Universal Intelligence", describing it as a large library containing every

thought, word, concept or action ever experienced by anyone. As I stared out the window,

I pondered the concept. Then it came to me. What if this Universal Intelligence was a

vast yet single mind? What if you could simply ask it questions, and it would supply you

with profound answers? Life changing insights that could guide you and anyone else you

shared them with. I decided to put that theory to a test.

I unfolded my legs, sat up in my chair, and laid my hands palm up in my lap. Breathing in through my nose and out through my mouth. With my eyes closed, I visualized a swirling ball of white light floating in the darkness. I saw the ball come closer and closer to me, until it was right in front of me and 8 feet tall. In my mind's eye I walked into the whirling sphere of light and felt exhilarated by the nearly limitless knowledge it held. As it spun around me, I asked a question. "What is the world loosing site of?"

I stood quietly for what seemed hours until a deep and subtle voice said the following words.

"I live and exist on all planes,

in all times, as all life,

with all possibilities at once.

I live in the courageous and the cowardly alike.

My light reveals kinship to the universe.

I am the friend you avoid,

and the stranger you know.

I am love.

Let me come home."

Since then, I've used this technique to channel through numerous writings. Here are some that I'd be honored to share with you.

"Pointing the Finger"

They say it's not polite to point.

Do you know where that came from?

Well, think about it.

When someone points at you,

You can actually feel it as well as see it.

Is there something more here than meets the eye?

Before the birth of Christ, there was a small yet prosperous

Village at the foothills of the Himalayas. The people of the

Village were so connected with nature and each other that

They grew to understand one simple fact. "To respect others

is to respect yourself because there is no difference." This

belief included animals, plants, and all other elements of

nature. Their connectedness gave them the opportunity to

enjoy great health and abundance. When one of their people

would get injured they were brought to a bed of reeds that

was conspicuously placed in the center of the village square.

All of the villagers would drop what they were doing and

assemble in a large circle around their wounded friend. When

every last member of the community was present in the square,

they would all lift their right hands & and point at the one

on the bed of reeds. Soon after, they lifted their left hands in the air. Their palms faced the sky. They pointed and smiled warmly at their friend. The wounded villager's body began to move as if it were being lovingly tickled by dozens of fingers, and the wounds would spontaneously heal. The villagers would go back to their chores with smiles, laughter and chatter. The healed villager would fall into a gentle sleep and wake cheerfully a few hours later.

One day a stonecutter from the village found a stranger wounded and unconscious in a quarry where he was gathering large stones for his next project. He gently lifted the man onto his stone cart, and headed back to the village. He laid the stranger onto the bed of reeds in the square and summoned the villagers. They came quickly. The fact that he was an outsider to the village didn't slow their response in the least. They began to point and smile at the wounded outsider. His body began to rise from the reeds and undulate. His eyes opened and were soon filled with fear. He looked around at the villagers. The closest one was 10 feet away, but he could feel all of their fingers moving around deep inside his body. His wounds spontaneously healed. He jumped to his feet and yelled, "Stop!" He ran up to the tall thin elderly villager who was standing closest to him. "What are you people doing to me!?", yelled the outsider to the man. "Healing your wounds", he replied calmly. The outsider turned to the crowd and shouted, "Where I come from I am a great ruler and I do not tolerate this type of evil in my kingdom or anywhere else my feet settle to the soil. I will return with an army to rid this land of your treachery!"

The army came and destroyed those who knew only love. In the ruler's kingdom, "Pointing" was outlawed. Three thousand years later it's just considered bad manners. Thru ought history, fear and ignorance have separated us from each other, nature & our own true potential.

We are turning the corner now.

The future is bright.

The adventure begins.

Remember who you are.

"Focus"

Ripping raging winds thru the canyon.

Explosive and unpredictable.

Path not clear, pattern undefined.

Take a wider look.

Perspective is the first step in attaining focus.

"Black Rain"

The silent falling of black rain.

Rain we tolerate. Rain we create.

Darkness amongst the city of light.

A driving torrent of anger, Forming puddles of grief.

We bathe in solitude.

Can a trillion points of lightlive in ignorance of each others existence?

Not for long. It won't be long now.

"Pain"

Catching the light, my memory burns bright.

Was it real. Is it real. Will I reveal the truth.

Urn to be one with the Earth and the Sun

And the Universe hands you more want.

Let down your guard. Don't think so hard.

Even in the darkest night,

You're still one with the light.

"Elements of Intention"

Ten steps on the path.

Turn, Turn, No Straight!

Warm wind to my back.

Cold darkness ahead.

The tunnel's deep, but inviting.

Warrior rising.

Stumble over those who have tried, yet failed.

Be present for the light.

It will come.

Be silent. Feel the hum.

The cobblestones begin to glow.

The path is clear.

You are, and have always been "The Path"

"Be Present"

Live not in the past or future

Miracles dwell where reality exists.

"Seeing"

How much of what we see is actually there?

How much of what's there do we actually see?

See sights, not thoughts.

Be love, not fear.

"Turn on the light"

Apprehension in the darkness. Hand on the light switch.

Turn on the light. Not yet. Please, not yet!

The darkness is warmed with sorrow. Anxious comfort.

I remember the light.

I was once burned by the sun's rays.

I remember that.

Is the switch jammed, or is my hand frozen? My arm grows heavy.

Must do it!......There!

No ceiling? No walls? No floor?!

I'm floating! I have wings.

I'm free.

I've always been free.

"The Prisoner"

The criminal went to trial,

Was found guilty,

Sentenced to life without parole;

But you're the one behind bars.

Learn to forgive,

And the governors pardon is on it's way.

"Face the fear of silence"

Run a mile a minute.

Life seems but a blur.

Faces fly bye in a whirr.

See nothing, but see it fast.

Feel nothing, but feel it fast.

Nothing exists, but speed.

Adrenalin without substance.

Trip, fall, get up.

Stand still.

Breath in the silence.

Each moment is now precious.

BE PRESENT.

There is no fear.

"The Lonely Vessel"

I walk the path.

I have no shadow.

There is no light.

I would share love, but there's only enough for me.

Even MY supplies are dwindling.

No light.

No love.

No existence.

He died of starvation at the kitchen table

Sitting next to a stocked refrigerator.

There is no receiving without giving,

and vis-versa.

"We create"

"Fate" is the reality that we allow others to create for us.

When you actively embrace your role as "Creator",

there is no fate.

Face it now, or embrace the lie.

Recognize your decisions.

"And"

Do we live in the hearts of others,

or do all hearts beat as one?

Do actions and events create icons,

or do icons create as well?

In a universe of "ORs" wall protect and imprison.

We reside in a universe of "ANDs".

We are powerful.

We are love.

Chapter Nine
Five Years Later

For the last 5 years I haven't written a word. I've put on 30 pounds. My blood pressure, cholesterol, and blood sugar have all risen. I'm stressed out, depressed, and generally unhappy with my life. Over these past years I've transferred the computer file for this book from one computer to another; but have never opened it to resume writing. What the hell happened?!!!

I'm now 90 days away from my 48th birthday. I've recently hired a life coach by the name of Barbara George who seems to possess the life experience, common sense, and coaching ability needed to get me back on track. Two weeks ago I sent her an electronic copy of my book to this point, with an outline of unfinished chapters. She red it, and at last week's session told me that it was a "Great Read", "Original" and "Very Touching". "People need to read this book", "You've got to make this your focus", and "When do you plan on having this finished by?" were a few of her statements and questions. I respected her opinion, So I scheduled time to open the "Angel.Doc" file on my computer's desktop, and begin writing.....Again.

It's a chilly and windy fall evening. I'm sitting in a quiet Coffee shop off Route 17 South in Paramus, New Jersey. I've just completed rereading my first seven chapters and the outline of chapters yet to be written. Dozens of questions and thoughts are now running through my head. "What happened to the person who wrote this book?", "There's lots of great insight and techniques for change that I could use to turn things back around in my life", "How could I write a "how to" book like this if I've fallen so far from grace?", "This book is like a time capsule that was buried and rediscovered to remind me of what's really important, and how to get back my wings". "Enough!!" I sprang to my feet, almost knocking my laptop computer on the floor. I quickly packed up my things and ran to my car in the empty parking lot behind the coffee shop. I rummaged through the files in the trunk of my car to find copies of a few of the forms I described in the book. With a number two pencil, a blank legal pad, and a few of my forms I camped out in the front seat of my car, and began to work. I was going to turn things around, and I knew just how to do it.

Chapter Ten
Ten Weeks Later

After numerous "Intention Action Outcome Journals", consultations with Jeffrey Tyler, three weeks of intensive media detox and some dietary changes; I had lost 26 pounds, significantly lowered my blood pressure, cholesterol and blood sugar levels. For the past two weeks I've been waking each morning with a sense of anticipation and optimism that's almost intoxicating. My friends, family and business associates have all been asking, "What have you been doing? You look ten years younger. You're glowing." I respond with a simple "Thank You", and a confident smile. The angel in my mirror has a twinkle in his eye. My old friend. I can see you clearly now.

Like my mom used to say, "When the challenges of life seem insurmountable, the real hero's don't measure themselves by the number of times they fall off the horse, but instead, the number of times they dust their pants off and get back on."

Be kind to yourself,

and always keep your eyes on the angel.

Form #101:

Past/Present/Future Worksheet

PAST	PRESENT	FUTURE
卌 卌 卌 卌 卌 卌 |||	||	卌 卌 卌 卌 卌 ||

Form #102:
Intention Action Outcome Journal (IAOJ)

INTENTION	ACTION	OUTCOME
Told my sons that I would create the most amazing sleep over birthday party in the backyard for them and 10 of their friends. DUE: 6/30	- Built a 10 foot screen & projected the movies and video games onto it. Attached to garage. Set up speakers and LCD projector. Also set up tuner and CD player for music. - Purchased 10 foot enclosed trampoline and set up in driveway. - Got 6 laser tag sets and planned out where we played. - Purchased 16 foot by 10 foot tent that the kids slept over in. - Purchased 9 three foot latex balloons. Rented a large tank of helium. Filled them up. Attached them to each other & added lights to create a UFO that we flew at 1000 feet. - Fed them pizza, popcorn, hot dogs, and soda.	- ME: "I had a great night with the kids and they were always surprised by each activity I planned. I really came through!!!!" - Stevie (My son): He gave me a 5 minute hug the next morning, and didn't stop smiling for two days. - Jeffrey (My son): Laughed and giggled all night long. - The Other Kids: All said, "This was the best party we ever went to!!!"

Made in the USA
Middletown, DE
06 October 2020

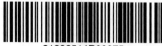